Weight Watchers™ Family Favourites

Sue Ashworth

SIMON & SCHUSTER
A VIACOM COMPANY

First published in Great Britain by Simon & Schuster, 1996
A Viacom Company

Copyright © 1996, Weight Watchers (UK) Ltd

Simon & Schuster Ltd
West Garden Place
Kendal Street
London W2 2AQ

Weight Watchers is the registered trademark of Weight Watchers International, Inc
and is used under its control by the publisher.

Design: Green Moore Lowenhoff
Typesetting: Stylize
Photography: Karl Adamson
Styling: Maria Kelly
Food preparation: Kathryn Hawkins

Weight Watchers Publications Manager: Juliet Hudson
Weight Watchers Publications Assistant: Celia Whiston

A CIP catalogue record is available from the British Library

ISBN 0-68481-662-8

Printed and bound in Italy by Rotolito Lombarda S.p.A.

Pictured on the front cover: *Toad-in-the-hole (page 38)*

Pictured on the back cover: *Summer Pudding and Lemon Meringues (page 74)*

Recipe notes:
Egg size is medium (size 3), unless otherwise stated.
Vegetables are medium-sized, unless otherwise stated.
It is important to use proper measuring spoons, not cutlery, for spoon measures.
1 tablespoon = 15 ml; 1 teaspoon = 5 ml.
Dried herbs can be substituted for fresh ones, but the flavour may not always
be as good. Halve the fresh-herb quantity stated in the recipe.

Vegetarian recipes:
These symbols show which recipes are suitable for vegetarians.

Ⓥ shows the recipe is vegetarian

V shows the recipe has a vegetarian option

Contents

Introduction

Here it is – the Weight Watchers book that you've been waiting for! *Family Favourites* is a cookery bible with your favourite recipes slimmed down to fit into a healthy, balanced diet. No longer do you need to forego that tempting portion of lasagne, coq au vin, or even fish and chips. Instead, you can make slim-line versions which fit in happily with your Weight Watchers Programme. The ingredients and cooking methods have been cleverly adjusted to reduce both fat and Calories – without reducing the taste! You'll even find recipes for luscious desserts that taste remarkably indulgent, but are far more innocent than their high-Calorie cousins. Time and time again you'll pick up this ingenious cookbook to remind yourself of the many ways that you can eat familiar favourites without piling on extra pounds. You'll be able to serve delicious meals to your family and friends without them guessing how light and healthy the food actually is! All of the recipes indicate Calories per serving and for those of you following the Weight Watchers 1,2,3 Success Programme, we've included Points as well. The 1,2,3 Success Programme has been devised by Weight Watchers to give you a quick way of seeing how light and healthy different foods actually are. Each food is allocated a number of Points, depending on how many Calories and grams of saturated fat it contains. To lose weight, you simply have to stick to a daily Point limit. As well as watching the pounds drop off, you'll know that you're eating a healthy diet, low in saturated fats. All you have to do is add up your daily Points. Your daily Point total will depend on whether you're male or female, what age you are, and how much you weigh. You can earn extra Points if you exercise, and when you have a special occasion coming up, you can save some of your Points for the big day. Your Weight Watchers Leader will be able to tell you how many Points you can have per day, and all about how to save and earn extra Points. Using the Point system to lose weight allows you real flexibility to eat the foods you love when you want to. You'll find that for everyday eating you'll automatically steer clear of foods that aren't so healthy because they'll cost you more Points. However, you won't feel guilty when you do eat the odd fatty or sugary treat, because you can simply treat it like any other food and count the Points. If you haven't yet started using the new Point system, ask your Weight Watchers Leader for a copy of our new 1,2,3 Success Programme, and get going on the most flexible diet ever. And take comfort in this wonderful new recipe book – it will help you on your way to healthy cooking and eating, Weight Watchers style!

Soups

In this short chapter you'll find four fabulous recipes for tasty, warming soups – recipes that will become firm favourites whether you're dieting or not! These recipes are so quick and simple to prepare they are virtually as easy to make as opening a can of soup, but they are worlds apart in terms of flavour. So get out that cooking pot and start your own soup kitchen – you'll be delighted that you did!

Minestrone Soup

Serves 4

Preparation time: 10 minutes
Cooking time: 30 minutes
Calories per serving: 220

Freezing: recommended

Enjoy the Italian influence of this delicious and quick-to-make soup.

1 tablespoon olive or
   vegetable oil
1 large onion, chopped
1 garlic clove, crushed
1 large carrot, sliced
3 oz (90 g) green beans, sliced
14 oz (420 g) canned chopped
   tomatoes
12 oz (360 g) canned haricot
   beans, rinsed and drained
1½ pints (900 ml) vegetable
   stock
2 oz (60 g) small pasta shapes
2 teaspoons dried mixed Italian
   herbs
salt and freshly ground black
   pepper

1. Heat the oil in a large saucepan. Add the onion and garlic and sauté gently for 5 minutes.
2. Add the carrot, green beans, tomatoes, haricot beans and vegetable stock. Bring to the boil, and then cover and reduce the heat. Simmer for 10–15 minutes.
3. Add the pasta and herbs and cook for about 8 minutes more, or until the pasta is cooked.
4. Season to taste with salt and pepper and serve in warm bowls.

Points per serving: 2.5
Total Points per recipe: 10

Cock-a-Leekie Soup

Serves 4

Preparation time: 15 minutes
Cooking time: 35 minutes
Calories per serving: 110

Freezing: recommended

Fresh chicken, leeks and onion make this superb Scottish soup.

1 tablespoon margarine
1 onion, chopped finely
2 leeks, sliced finely
8 oz (240 g) raw chicken leg,
   skinned
1½ pints (900 ml) water
1 tablespoon chopped fresh
   parsley
salt and freshly ground black
   pepper

1. Melt the margarine in a large saucepan and gently sauté the onion and leeks for about 10 minutes, until softened.
2. Add the chicken to the saucepan with the water. Bring to the boil and then reduce the heat. Cover and simmer gently for 20 minutes.
3. Remove the chicken from the saucepan, using a draining spoon, and place on a chopping board. Allow to cool slightly, and then remove all the meat and discard the bone. Chop the meat and return it to the saucepan with the parsley.
4. Reheat the soup and season to taste with salt and pepper. Serve at once in warm soup bowls.

Points per serving: 2
Total Points per recipe: 8

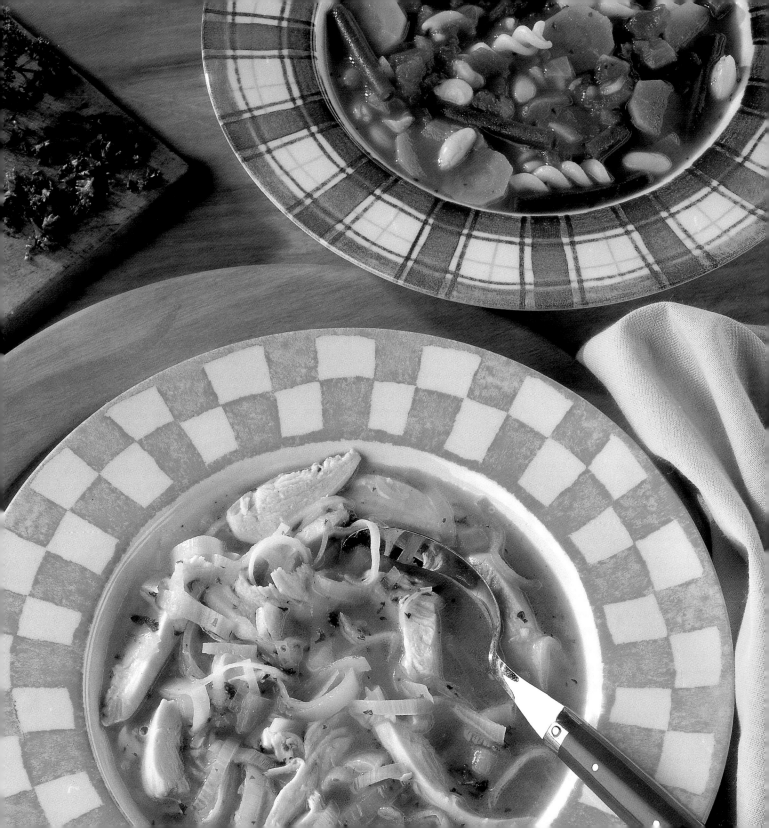

Tomato Soup

Serves 4

Preparation time: 5 minutes
Cooking time: 25 minutes
Calories per serving: 120

Freezing: recommended

Use canned tomatoes for speed and convenience in this excellent home-made favourite.

1 tablespoon vegetable oil
1 large onion, chopped
14 oz (420 g) canned tomatoes
2 tablespoons tomato purée
³/₄ pint (450 ml) vegetable stock
2 tablespoons cornflour
¹/₂ pint (300 ml) skimmed milk
salt and freshly ground black pepper

1. Heat the oil in a large saucepan. Add the onion and sauté gently for 5 minutes.
2. Add the tomatoes, tomato purée and stock. Bring to the boil, and then cover and simmer gently for 15 minutes.
3. Transfer to a liquidiser or food processor, and blend for about 15 seconds, or until smooth. Return to the saucepan.
4. Blend the cornflour to a smooth paste with 3–4 tablespoons of the milk, and then add it to the saucepan with the remaining milk. Heat, stirring constantly, until the soup is thickened and smooth.
5. Season to taste with salt and pepper, and serve piping hot in warm soup bowls.

Points per serving: 1.5
Total Points per recipe: 6

Leek and Potato Soup

Serves 4

Preparation time: 15 minutes
Cooking time: 35 minutes
Calories per serving: 165

Freezing: recommended

Serve this thick, warming soup piping hot on a cold winter's day.

1 lb (480 g) leeks, chopped finely
1 lb (480 g) potatoes, peeled and chopped
2 tablespoons chopped fresh parsley + extra to garnish
1¹/₂ pints (900 ml) vegetable stock
¹/₄ pint (150 ml) skimmed milk
salt and freshly ground black pepper

1 tablespoon margarine
1 onion, chopped finely

1. Melt the margarine in a large saucepan and gently sauté the onion and leeks for about 10 minutes, until softened.
2. Add the potatoes, parsley and stock. Bring to the boil and then cover and reduce the heat. Simmer gently for about 20 minutes, or until the vegetables are tender.
3. Add the milk to the saucepan and gently reheat. Season to taste with salt and pepper and serve piping hot in warm soup bowls, sprinkled with extra chopped parsley.

Cook's note:
Blend the soup in a liquidiser or food processor to make it extra smooth.

Points per serving: 2
Total Points per recipe: 8

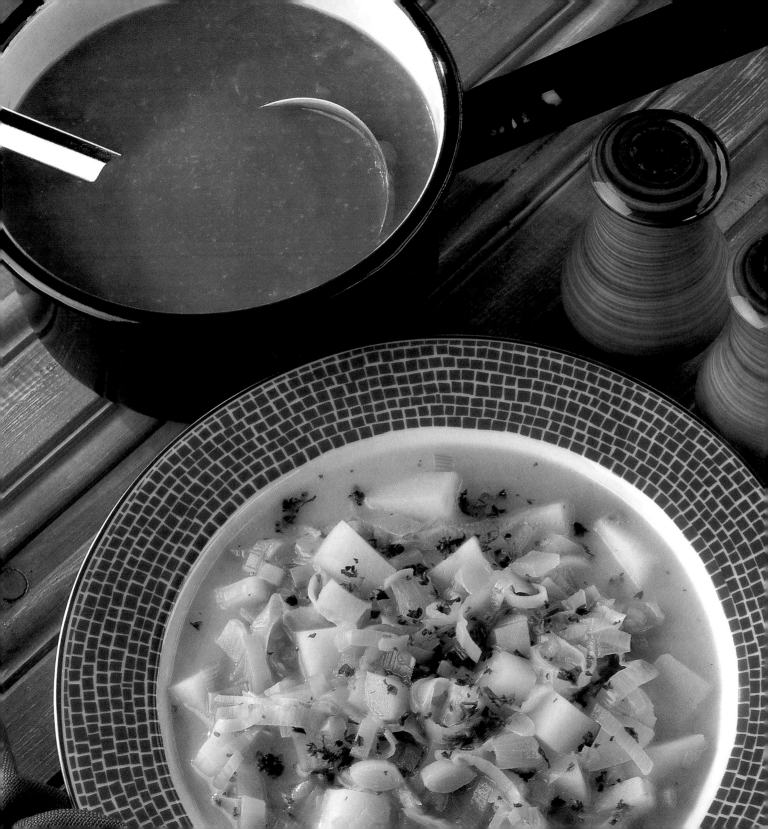

Pasta

Pasta dishes are so firmly established as some of our best-loved recipes, it's a wonder how we ever lived without them! The perfect food for modern-day living, pasta is quick to prepare, inexpensive and loved by everyone – including those of us who are watching our weight! This is no bad thing, as pasta is a basic carbohydrate food – a great source of energy to build a meal around. However, pasta recipes can quickly become heavy and Calorie-laden when served with rich sauces. Luckily, this chapter gives some bright ideas for adapting classic pasta dishes into lighter versions that will sit comfortably in our diets – and on our hips!

Macaroni Cheese

Serves 4

Preparation time: 10 minutes
Cooking time: 20 minutes
Calories per serving: 395

Freezing: recommended

V If using vegetarian cheese

Cheap, cheerful and satisfying – no wonder this dish is always a welcome family meal!

6 oz (180 g) macaroni
2 tablespoons margarine
1½ oz (45 g) plain flour
¾ pint (450 ml) skimmed milk
6 oz (180 g) reduced-fat Cheddar cheese
½ oz (15 g) dried breadcrumbs
salt and cayenne pepper

1. Cook the macaroni in plenty of lightly salted boiling water for about 10 minutes, or until just tender.
2. Meanwhile, heat the margarine, flour and milk in a saucepan, stirring constantly with a small whisk, until the sauce boils and thickens. Cook for 1 minute, and then remove from the heat. Preheat the grill.
3. Stir about two-thirds of the cheese into the sauce, and then season with salt and cayenne pepper. Drain the macaroni thoroughly and stir it into the sauce. Transfer the mixture to a 3-pint (2-litre) heatproof dish.
4. Sprinkle the breadcrumbs and remaining cheese over the surface of the dish, and then grill until browned and bubbling.

Points per serving: 7.5
Total Points per recipe: 30

Tuna Pasta Supper

Serves 4

Preparation time: 15 minutes
Cooking time: 50 minutes
Calories per serving: 350

Freezing: not recommended

Whizz together this tasty supper dish in no time at all, and then reap the compliments!

4 oz (120 g) pasta shapes
12 oz (360 g) broccoli florets
1 teaspoon margarine
7 oz (210 g) canned tuna in brine, drained
2 eggs
¾ pint (450 ml) skimmed milk
3 oz (90 g) Red Leicester cheese, grated
salt and freshly ground black pepper

1. Cook the pasta shapes in plenty of lightly salted boiling water for about 8–10 minutes, or until just tender. Drain and rinse with cold water.
2. Meanwhile, cook the broccoli for 5–6 minutes in a little lightly salted boiling water, until tender. Drain well.
3. Preheat the oven to Gas Mark 5/190°C/375°F. Grease a 3-pint (2-litre) ovenproof dish with the margarine. Put the cooked pasta and broccoli into the dish. Flake the tuna fish and scatter it over the top.
4. Beat together the eggs and milk, and stir in most of the cheese. Season well with salt and pepper, and then pour into the dish. Sprinkle the remaining cheese over the top.
5. Bake for 40 minutes, or until set and golden brown.

Points per serving: 6
Total Points per recipe: 24

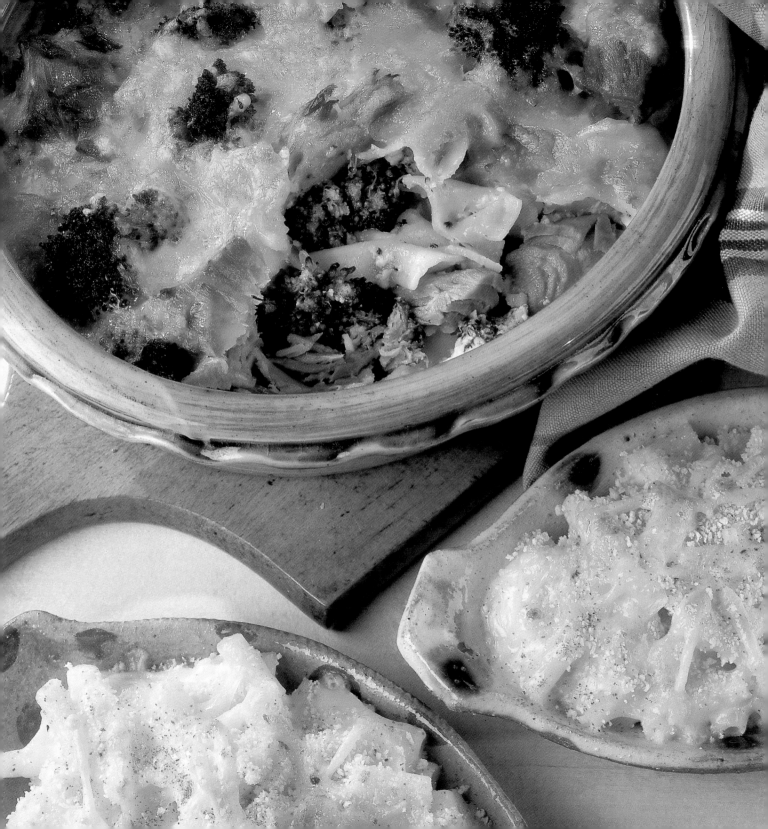

Spaghetti Carbonara

Serves 4

Preparation time: 10 minutes
Cooking time: 15 minutes
Calories per serving: 400

Freezing: not recommended

V

Use pasta shapes instead of spaghetti in this dish, if you prefer.

8 oz (240 g) spaghetti or
  pasta shapes
2 teaspoons margarine
1 small onion, chopped finely
1 garlic clove, peeled and left
  whole
6 oz (180 g) low-fat soft cheese
2 eggs
¼ pint (150 ml) skimmed milk
2 oz (60 g) Parma ham or lean
  boiled ham, cut in strips
1 oz (30 g) parmesan cheese,
  grated finely
1 tablespoon chopped fresh
  oregano or parsley
salt and freshly ground black
  pepper
sprigs of fresh oregano or
  parsley, to garnish

1. Bring a large saucepan of lightly salted water to the boil. Add the spaghetti or pasta shapes and cook for about 8 minutes, or until just tender – *al dente*. Check the pack instructions for exact timings.
2. Meanwhile, melt the margarine in a frying pan and sauté the onion and garlic clove for about 5 minutes, until softened. Discard the garlic clove.
3. Put the soft cheese into a large mixing bowl and beat it with a wooden spoon until soft. Stir in the eggs and cooked onion, mixing until combined. Add the milk, ham, most of the parmesan, and the oregano or parsley. Season with salt and pepper.
4. Drain the spaghetti or pasta shapes and return to the saucepan, stirring in the carbonara mixture. Heat gently for about 2 minutes, stirring until the mixture has thickened.
5. Divide the pasta between 4 warm serving plates. Sprinkle with the remaining parmesan, and garnish with sprigs of oregano or parsley. Serve at once.

Points per serving: 7
Total Points per recipe: 28

V Vegetarian option:
Omit the ham. This will reduce the Points per serving to 6 and the Total Points per recipe to 24.

Spaghetti Bolognese

Serves 4

Preparation time: 15 minutes
Cooking time: 35 minutes
Calories per serving: 495

Freezing: recommended for bolognese sauce

V

An all-time favourite – and why not? It still tastes as good as ever!

12 oz (360 g) extra-lean
  minced beef
1 large onion, chopped finely
2 garlic cloves, crushed
  (optional)
2 celery sticks, sliced
1 large carrot, chopped
14 oz (420 g) canned chopped
  tomatoes
8 oz (240 g) mushrooms, wiped
  and sliced
1 teaspoon dried mixed Italian
  herbs
1 tablespoon tomato purée
8 oz (240 g) quick-cook
  spaghetti
salt and freshly ground black
  pepper
4 teaspoons grated parmesan
  cheese

1. Dry-fry the minced beef in a large non-stick saucepan until browned.
2. Add the onion and garlic, if using, and cook for 4–5 minutes, or until softened. Add the celery and carrot and cook for 2 minutes more.
3. Add the canned tomatoes, mushrooms, herbs and tomato purée. Stir well and then bring to the boil. Cover and reduce the heat. Simmer gently for 10 minutes and then remove the lid and cook for 15 minutes more.
4. Meanwhile, cook the spaghetti in plenty of lightly salted boiling water, according to pack instructions.
5. Check the seasoning, and add salt and pepper to taste. Drain the spaghetti, divide between 4 warm serving plates and top with the bolognese sauce. Sprinkle 1 teaspoon of grated parmesan on to each portion and serve at once.

Points per serving: 6
Total Points per recipe: 24

V Vegetarian option:
Substitute 9 oz (270 g) reconstituted soya mince for the minced beef. This will reduce the Points per serving to 4.5 and the Total Points per recipe to 18.

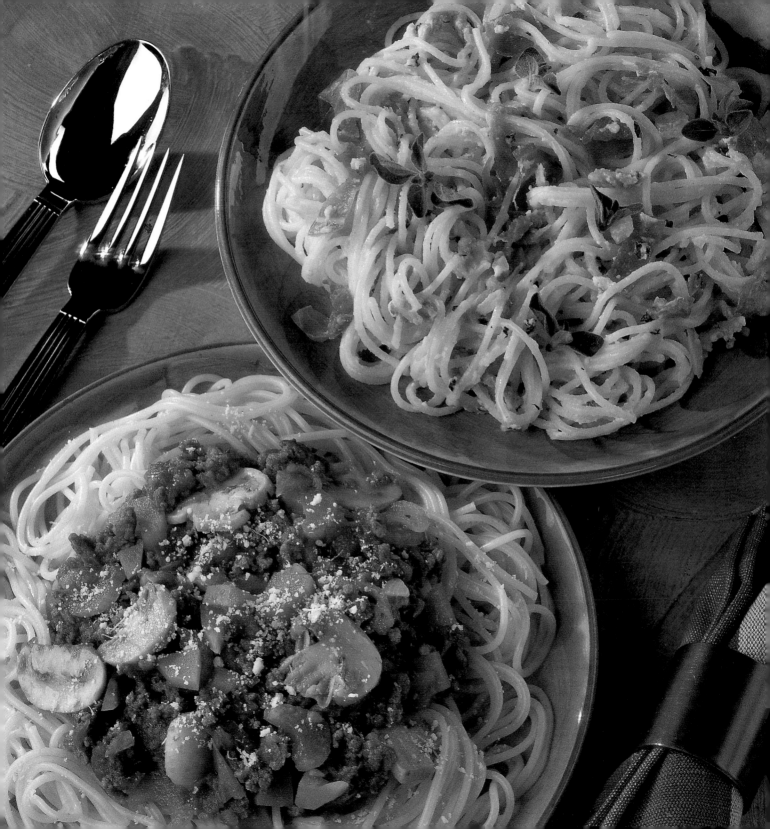

Cannelloni

Serves 4

Preparation time: 40 minutes
Cooking time: 1 hour
Calories per serving: 430

Freezing: recommended

Ⓥ If using vegetarian cheese

These large pasta tubes are
filled with a spinach and
soft cheese mixture, and
then baked with a delicious
tomato sauce.

1 lb (480 g) fresh spinach
8 oz (240 g) low-fat soft cheese
  with garlic and herbs
8 oz (240 g) cannelloni tubes
1 tablespoon olive oil
1 onion, chopped finely
14 oz (420 g) canned chopped
  tomatoes
1 tablespoon tomato purée
1 teaspoon mixed dried Italian
  herbs
2 oz (60 g) parmesan cheese,
  grated finely
salt and freshly ground black
  pepper

1. Wash the spinach thoroughly and place it in a very large saucepan. Cover and cook over a low heat for about 6 minutes, until the spinach has wilted (no extra water is needed). Drain well, squeezing out the excess moisture using the back of a wooden spoon. Cool and chop finely.
2. Mix together the chopped spinach and the soft cheese, and season well with salt and pepper.
3. Cook the cannelloni tubes in a large saucepan of lightly salted boiling water for about 12 minutes, until just tender. (Check the pack instructions for exact timings.) Drain, cool slightly, and then fill with the spinach mixture. Lightly grease a shallow ovenproof dish with a little of the olive oil and then arrange the cannelloni in the baking dish.
4. Preheat the oven to Gas Mark 4/180°C/350°F.
5. Heat the remaining olive oil in a saucepan and sauté the onion for about 3 minutes, until softened. Add the tomatoes, tomato purée and herbs. Cook, uncovered, for about 10 minutes. Season with salt and pepper and then pour over the cannelloni. Sprinkle with half the parmesan.
6. Bake for 25–30 minutes, until bubbling and browned. Serve at once, sprinkled with the remaining parmesan.

Points per serving: 7
Total Points per recipe: 28

Cook's note:
Frozen or canned spinach can be used if fresh is not available.

Lasagne

Serves 4

Preparation time: 25 minutes
Cooking time: 1 hour
Calories per serving: 480

Freezing: recommended

V

For convenience, choose
lasagne sheets that do not
need pre-cooking.

12 oz (360 g) extra-lean
  minced beef
1 onion, chopped
1 garlic clove, crushed

6 oz (180 g) mushrooms, wiped
  and sliced
14 oz (420 g) canned chopped
  tomatoes
¼ pint (150 ml) vegetable stock
½ teaspoon dried mixed Italian
  herbs
4 oz (120 g) no pre-cook lasagne
  sheets
salt and freshly ground black
  pepper
For the cheese sauce:
½ pint (300 ml) skimmed milk
3 tablespoons plain white flour
1 tablespoon margarine
2 oz (60 g) mature Cheddar
  cheese, grated

1. Dry-fry the minced beef in a large non-stick saucepan until browned, stirring to break it up well. Add the onion and garlic. Cook for about 3 minutes, or until softened. Add the mushrooms, tomatoes, stock and herbs. Bring to the boil and then reduce the heat and simmer for 15–20 minutes, until slightly thickened. Season to taste and remove from the heat.
2. Preheat the oven to Gas Mark 5/190°C/375°F.
3. To make the cheese sauce, heat the milk, flour and margarine in a saucepan, stirring constantly with a small wire whisk, until thickened and smooth. Remove from the heat and add most of the cheese. Season to taste with salt and pepper.
4. Spoon half the beef mixture into an oblong ovenproof dish and layer half the lasagne sheets over the top. Spread 2–3 tablespoons of cheese sauce over the lasagne, and then the rest of the meat mixture. Cover with the remaining lasagne sheets and pour the rest of the cheese sauce over the top. Sprinkle with the remaining grated cheese and bake for 50–60 minutes, until golden brown and bubbling.

Points per serving: 7
Total Points per recipe: 28

V Vegetarian option:
Substitute 9 oz (270 g) of reconstituted soya mince for the beef. This will reduce the Points per serving to 6 and the Total Points per recipe to 24.

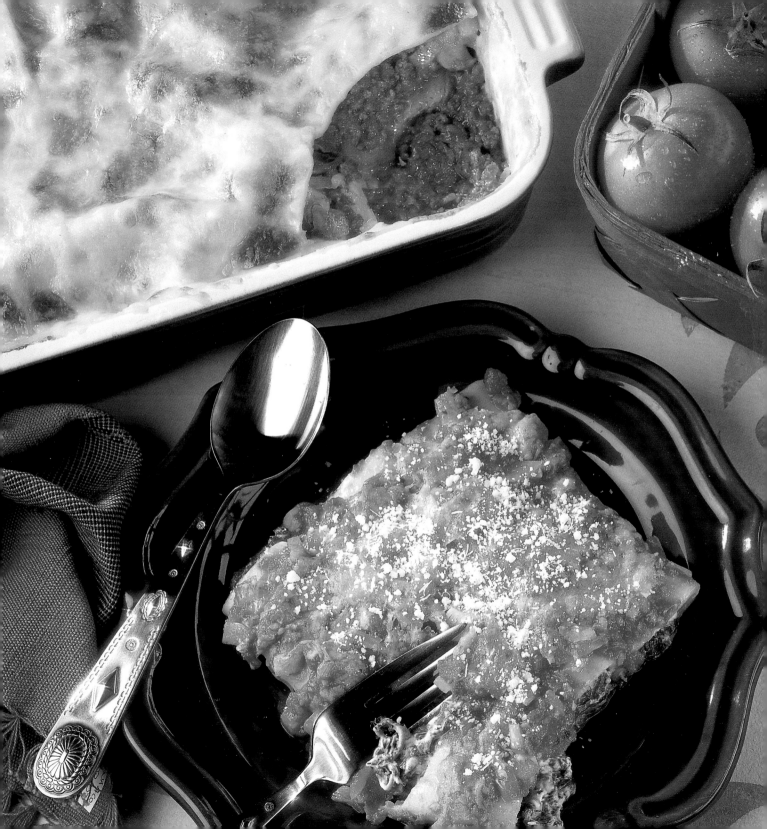

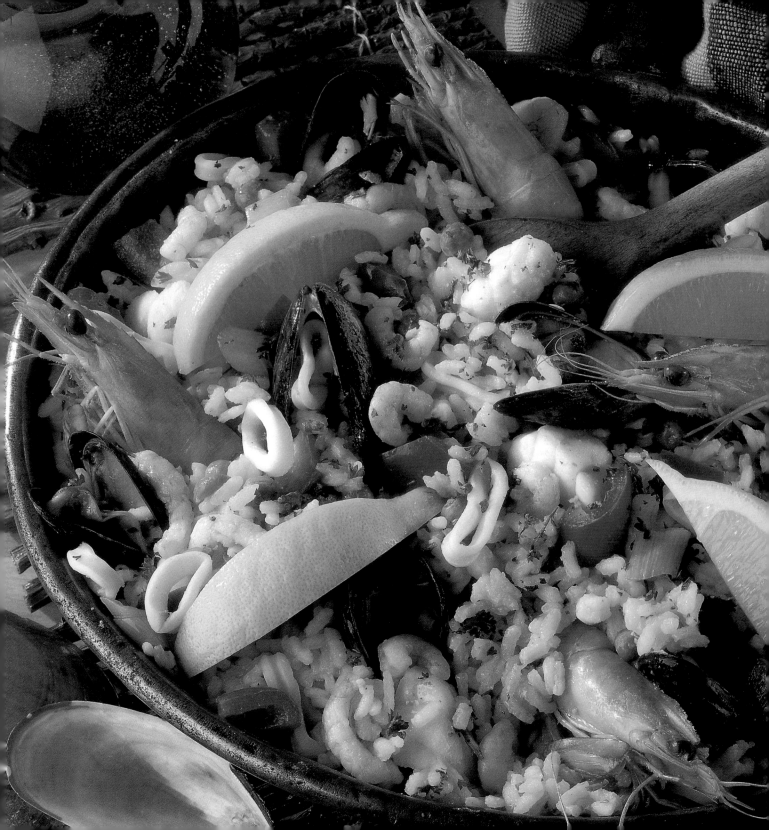

Fish

Low in fat and high in flavour, fish is the perfect choice for healthy eating. Yet so many of our favourite fish recipes are high in fat and Calories because of the way they are cooked – traditional fish and chips is undoubtedly the best (or worst) example. So how do you take advantage of the delicious flavour of fish without ruining your diet? Just replace some of the high-Calorie ingredients with lower-Calorie alternatives. Cut out the fat and choose lighter cooking methods, and your meals will be much healthier. So trawl your way through the recipe suggestions in this chapter – you certainly won't have to fish for compliments at *your* mealtimes!

Paella

Serves 6

Preparation time: 20 minutes
Cooking time: 50 minutes
Calories per serving: 475

Freezing: not recommended

This fabulous seafood medley will remind you of holidays abroad. Enjoy the memories!

2½ pints (1.5 litres) fish or chicken stock
1 small onion, halved
a pinch of saffron strands (optional)
2 tablespoons olive oil
2 garlic cloves, crushed
a bunch of spring onions, chopped finely
1 red pepper, de-seeded and chopped

1 lb (480 g) risotto rice
12 oz (360 g) firm white fish (e.g. monkfish, hake or cod), cut in large chunks
6 oz (180 g) squid rings
6 oz (180 g) prawns in shells
6 oz (180 g) fresh mussels, scrubbed (or canned, drained mussels)
6 oz (180 g) shrimps, shelled
2 tablespoons chopped fresh parsley
1 bay leaf
4 fl oz (120 ml) dry white wine
1 tablespoon lemon juice
2 oz (60 g) frozen peas
salt and freshly ground black pepper
lemon wedges and chopped fresh parsley, to garnish

4. Add the remaining ingredients (except for seasoning), stirring well. Cook gently for about 20 minutes, stirring occasionally. Add extra liquid, if needed.
5. Discard any fresh mussels that have not opened. Season the paella well with salt and pepper, and then garnish with lemon wedges and parsley and serve at once.

Points per serving: 7.5
Total Points per recipe: 45

1. Heat the stock with the onion and saffron (if using) in a medium-sized saucepan. Cover and simmer for 10–15 minutes. Strain the stock, discarding the onion.
2. Meanwhile, heat the oil in a wok or large frying pan, and add the garlic, spring onions and red pepper. Sauté for about 5 minutes, or until softened.
3. Stir the rice into the pan and sauté for 2–3 minutes. Pour in the hot strained stock and bring to the boil. Reduce the heat and simmer gently for 10 minutes.

Prawn Cocktail

Serves 4

Preparation time: 10 minutes
Calories per serving: 90

Freezing: not recommended

**Britain's favourite starter gets
the low-Calorie treatment!**

2 teaspoons tomato purée
4 teaspoons low-Calorie
   mayonnaise

5 fl oz (150 ml) low-fat natural
   yogurt
8 oz (240 g) peeled prawns,
   thawed if frozen
1 teaspoon lemon juice
salt and freshly ground black
   pepper
shredded lettuce, to serve
sprigs of parsley and lemon
   wedges, to garnish

1. Mix together the tomato purée and mayonnaise. Add the yogurt
and stir well until blended.
2. Gently mix the prawns into the dressing. Add the lemon juice
and season with salt and pepper.
3. Arrange the lettuce in the base of 4 serving dishes or glasses,
and then divide the prawns and dressing between the dishes.
Serve at once, garnished with sprigs of parsley and lemon wedges.

Points per serving: 1.5
Total Points per recipe: 6

Cod Mornay

Serves 4

Preparation and cooking time:
20 minutes
Calories per serving: 250

Freezing: not recommended

**A well-flavoured cheese sauce
perfectly complements cod
or any other white fish.**

4 × 6 oz (180 g) cod fillets
1 bay leaf

¼ pint (150 ml) skimmed milk
1 tablespoon margarine
2 tablespoons plain white flour
1 oz (30 g) Gruyère cheese,
   grated finely
1 oz (30 g) parmesan cheese,
   grated finely
½ teaspoon French mustard
salt and freshly ground black
   pepper

1. Place the fish in a frying pan and add just enough cold water
to cover. Add the bay leaf. Heat gently and poach the fish for about
6–8 minutes, until the flesh is opaque and flakes easily.
2. Strain ¼ pint (150 ml) of the cooking liquid into a saucepan.
Transfer the fish to 4 serving plates and keep warm. Discard the
bay leaf and the remaining fish stock.
3. Add the milk, margarine and flour to the strained fish stock and
heat, stirring constantly with a small wire whisk, until thickened
and smooth. Cook for 1 minute, and then remove from the heat
and add the grated cheese and mustard. Season to taste.
4. Pour the sauce over the fish and serve at once.

Points per serving: 6
Total Points per recipe: 24

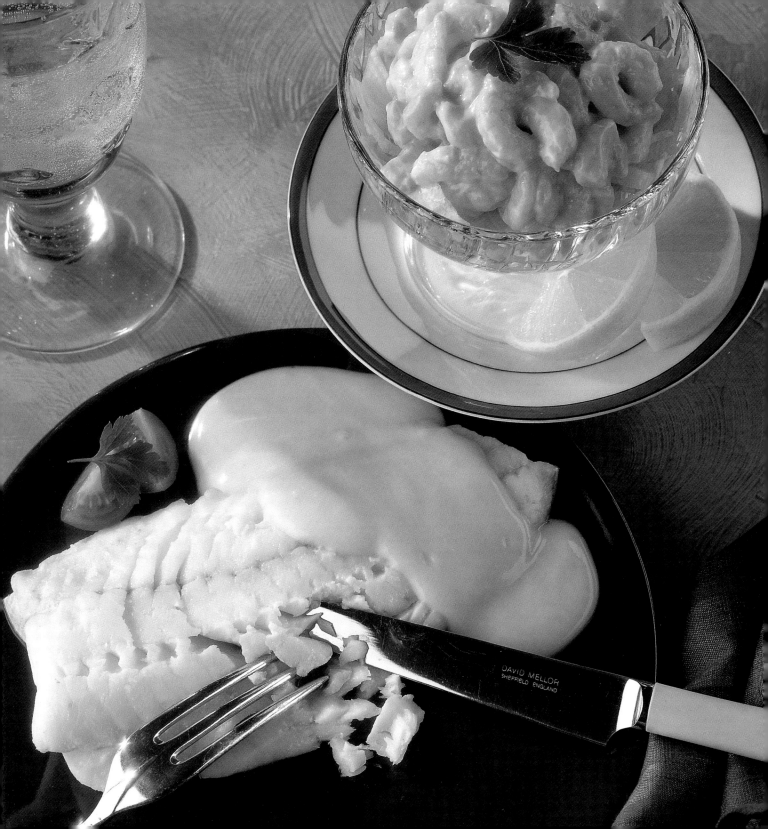

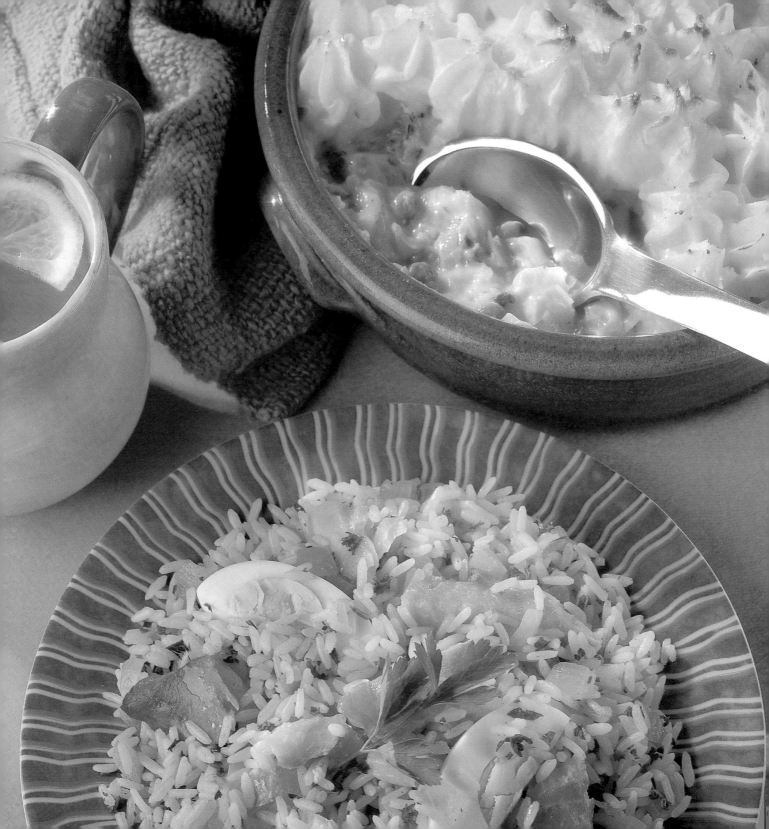

Kedgeree

Serves 4

Preparation time: 20 minutes
Cooking time: 20 minutes
Calories per serving: 345

Freezing: recommended

Smoked haddock or cod with
rice and spice makes a very
tasty meal.

1 lb (480 g) smoked cod
  or haddock fillet

1 tablespoon vegetable oil
6 oz (180 g) long-grain rice
1 onion, chopped
2 teaspoons curry powder
  (optional)
2 eggs, hard-boiled and
  quartered
1 tablespoon chopped fresh
  parsley
salt and freshly ground black
  pepper
fresh parsley, to garnish

1. Put the smoked fillet into a large frying pan and pour in enough cold water to just cover it. Poach gently for about 5 minutes, or until the fish is opaque and flakes easily. Remove the fish, discarding any skin and bones, and flake the flesh. Strain the cooking liquid into a measuring jug to make 1½ pints (900 ml), adding water if necessary.
2. Heat the oil in a frying pan and add the rice and onion. Sauté gently for about 5 minutes, and then add the curry powder (if using) and cook for 1 minute more.
3. Add the fish stock to the pan and bring to the boil. Reduce the heat and simmer, stirring occasionally, until the liquid is absorbed and the rice is cooked.
4. Add the poached fish, hard-boiled eggs and parsley to the saucepan. Season with salt and pepper. Heat through for 2–3 minutes, and then serve, garnished with fresh parsley.

Points per serving: 5
Total Points per recipe: 20

Fish Pie

Serves 4

Preparation time: 20 minutes
Cooking time: 1 hour 10
minutes
Calories per serving: 360

Freezing: recommended

Nutritious and economical,
this is an excellent meal for
the whole family.

1½ lb (720 g) potatoes
2 large leeks, chopped
½ pint (300 ml) + 2
  tablespoons skimmed milk
1 tablespoon chopped fresh
  parsley
1 oz (30 g) margarine
2 oz (60 g) plain flour
1 lb (480 g) skinned and boned
  cod, cut in chunks
1 oz (30 g) frozen peas
salt and freshly ground black
  pepper

1. Cook the potatoes in lightly salted boiling water until just tender. Meanwhile, cook the leeks in a little boiling water for about 5 minutes.
2. Drain the potatoes and leeks, reserving the cooking liquid. Mash the potatoes, adding 2 tablespoons of milk. Top the remaining ½ pint (300 ml) of milk up to ¾ pint (450 ml) with the cooking liquid from the potatoes and leeks. Stir in the parsley.
3. Heat the margarine, flour and milk mixture in a saucepan, stirring constantly with a small wire whisk, until thickened and smooth. Check the seasoning, adding salt and pepper if necessary.
4. Preheat the oven to Gas Mark 5/190°C/375°F.
5. Place the fish in a 2-pint (1.2-litre) baking dish, and scatter the cooked leeks and frozen peas on top. Pour over the parsley sauce and mix gently. Spoon the mashed potato over the top, roughing up the surface with a fork. Bake for 35–40 minutes, until cooked and lightly browned.

Points per serving: 6
Total Points per dish: 24

Fish and Chips

Serves 4

Preparation time: 15 minutes
Cooking time: 50 minutes
Calories per serving: 405

Freezing: not recommended

This oven-baked version of one of our best-loved supper dishes radically reduces its fat and Calorie content.

2 tablespoons vegetable oil
1½ lb (720 g) unpeeled potatoes, scrubbed and cut in wedges
4 × 6 oz (180 g) cod or haddock fillets
2 tablespoons plain white flour, seasoned
1 egg
2 oz (60 g) dried breadcrumbs
salt and freshly ground black pepper

1. Preheat the oven to Gas Mark 6/200°C/400°F. Grease a roasting pan and baking sheet with 1 teaspoon of the oil. Heat the roasting pan in the oven for 5 minutes.
2. Put the potato wedges in the roasting pan and brush them with the remaining oil. Sprinkle with salt, and then bake for about 30 minutes, or until barely tender. Reduce the oven temperature to Gas Mark 5/190°C/375°F.
3. Wash the fish fillets and pat them dry with kitchen paper. Sprinkle the seasoned flour on a plate, and dip the fish fillets into it to coat.
4. Beat the egg in a shallow bowl with 2 tablespoons of cold water. Sprinkle the breadcrumbs on another plate. Dip the floured fish fillets into the egg, and then coat with the breadcrumbs. Place the fillets on the prepared baking sheet and bake for 15–20 minutes, until the fish is cooked and the chips are golden brown.
5. Serve the fish with the oven-baked chips, seasoned to taste.

Points per serving: 7.5
Total Points per recipe: 30

Fishcakes

Serves 4

Preparation time: 20 minutes
Cooking time: 20 minutes
Calories per serving: 245

Freezing: recommended

This recipe uses cod fillet, but for speed you could substitute 10 oz (300 g) of canned tuna fish in brine, drained well.

12 oz (360 g) cod fillet
1 lb (480 g) cooked potato, mashed
1 tablespoon chopped fresh parsley or chives
4 tablespoons skimmed milk
1 egg
6 tablespoons dried breadcrumbs
salt and freshly ground black pepper

1. Preheat the oven to Gas Mark 5/190°C/375°F.
2. Poach the fish in a little water for about 6–8 minutes, until the flesh is opaque and flakes easily. Alternatively, place the fish on a microwave dish, cover and microwave on HIGH (100%) for 4–5 minutes. Allow to stand for 3–4 minutes, and then remove any skin and bones and flake the fish.
3. Mix the flaked fish with the mashed potato, parsley or chives and milk. Season with salt and pepper. Form into 8 round cakes.
4. Beat the egg with 2 tablespoons of water in a shallow bowl. Place the breadcrumbs in another dish.
5. Dip the fishcakes in the beaten egg and then coat with the breadcrumbs. Place on a non-stick baking sheet and bake for 20 minutes, until golden brown.

Points per serving: 4.5
Total Points per recipe: 18

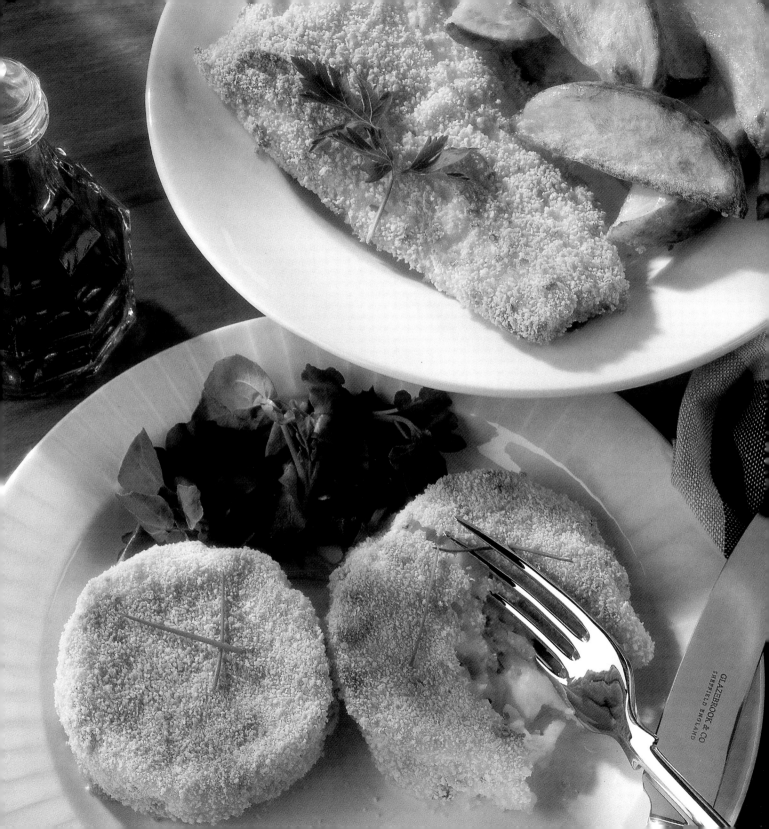

Chicken

Some classic chicken recipes appear in this chapter, from the longtime children's favourite, Chicken Nuggets, to the more sophisticated Chicken Supreme (both on page 33). All the recipes have been given the Weight Watchers treatment, which means they have been pared down Calorie-wise, but not in flavour. By using skinless chicken and cutting out high-fat extras, you can enjoy the same dishes you've always loved. As you work your way through the recipe ideas in this chapter you'll learn how to trim the fat, not the taste.

Coronation Chicken

Serves 4

Preparation time: 10 minutes
Calories per serving: 245

Freezing: not recommended

Cold chicken in a creamy, mild curry sauce is perfect for a summer's day.

5 fl oz (150 ml) low-fat natural yogurt
2 teaspoons mild curry powder
2 small bananas, sliced
2 oz (60 g) ready-to-eat dried apricots, chopped
1 oz (30 g) raisins or sultanas
12 oz (360 g) skinless, boneless cooked chicken, sliced
salt and freshly ground black pepper

1. Mix together the yogurt and curry powder in a large bowl.
2. Add the bananas, apricots, and raisins or sultanas. Mix in the chicken, stirring gently to coat with the curry sauce. Season to taste with salt and pepper.
3. Keep covered and refrigerated until ready to serve.

Points per serving: 4
Total Points per recipe: 16

Cook's note:
A few finely chopped fresh mint leaves will add to the taste of this delicious salad.

Chicken Casserole

Serves 4

Preparation time: 15 minutes
Cooking time: 1 hour 20 minutes
Calories per serving: 230

Freezing: recommended

Serve this chicken casserole with boiled or jacket potatoes, rice or pasta.

1 tablespoon vegetable oil
2 large leeks, sliced
2 celery sticks, sliced
2 carrots, chopped
1 onion, chopped
15 oz (450 g) skinless, boneless chicken, cut in large chunks
3/4 pint (450 ml) chicken stock
1 tablespoon chopped fresh parsley
1 bay leaf
1 tablespoon cornflour, blended with 2 tablespoons cold water
salt and freshly ground black pepper

1. Preheat the oven to Gas Mark 4/180°C/350°F.
2. Heat the oil in a large flameproof casserole and sauté the leeks, celery, carrots and onion for 3–4 minutes, until softened.
3. Add the chicken and cook until sealed all over. Stir in the stock, parsley and bay leaf, and season with salt and pepper.
4. Cover the casserole and transfer it to the oven. Cook for 1–1 1/4 hours.
5. Remove the bay leaf. Stir the blended cornflour into the casserole. Cook for 5 minutes more.
6. Serve the casserole on warm plates.

Selections per serving:
1/2 Fat; 3 Protein; 2 Vegetable; 20 Optional Calories

Points per serving: 3
Total Points per recipe: 12

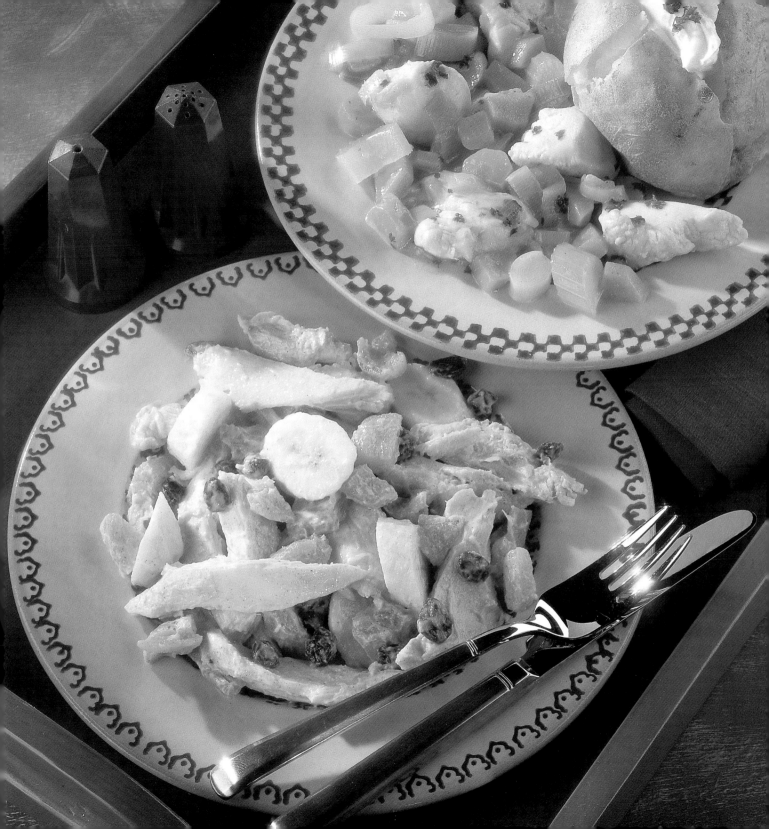

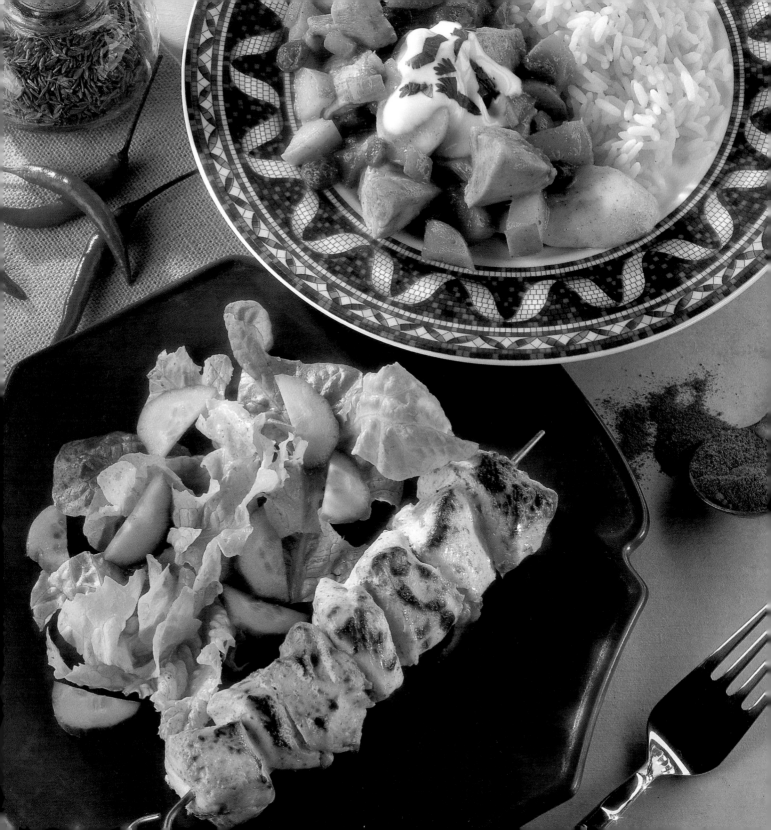

Chicken Curry

Serves 4

Preparation time: 10 minutes
Cooking time: 55 minutes
Calories per serving: 345

Freezing: recommended

Use mild, medium or hot curry powder according to your preference.

1 tablespoon vegetable oil
1 onion, chopped
1 medium-sized apple, chopped
2 tablespoons curry powder
12 oz (360 g) skinless, boneless chicken, cut in chunks
½ pint (300 ml) chicken stock
1 oz (30 g) sultanas
4 oz (120 g) long-grain rice
1 small banana, sliced
salt and freshly ground black pepper
4 tablespoons low-fat natural yogurt, to serve
chopped fresh coriander or parsley, to garnish

1. Heat the vegetable oil in a large saucepan and sauté the onion and apple for 3–4 minutes. Add the curry powder and cook, stirring, for 1 minute more.
2. Add the chicken to the saucepan and cook for 2–3 minutes, until sealed all over.
3. Add the chicken stock and sultanas to the saucepan. Bring to the boil, and then reduce the heat. Cover and simmer gently for about 40 minutes.
4. About 15 minutes before the end of cooking, cook the rice in plenty of lightly salted boiling water for about 12 minutes, or until tender. Drain thoroughly and rinse with boiling water.
5. Stir the banana into the curry. Check the seasoning and add salt and pepper to taste.
6. Serve the curry with the hot cooked rice. Spoon one tablespoon of yogurt on each portion and sprinkle with chopped fresh coriander or parsley.

Points per serving: 5
Total Points per recipe: 20

Chicken Tikka

Serves 6

Preparation time: 30 minutes + 3–4 hours marinating
Cooking time: 15 minutes
Calories per serving: 165

Freezing: not recommended

The secret of this superb recipe lies in leaving the chicken in the spicy marinade for several hours.

1 lb 6 oz (660 g) skinned and boned chicken, cubed
5 fl oz (150 ml) white vinegar
2 teaspoons salt
2 garlic cloves, crushed
2 teaspoons chilli powder
1 teaspoon finely grated fresh root ginger
1 teaspoon chopped fresh mint
½ teaspoon cumin seeds, crushed or ground cumin
1 tablespoon vegetable oil
5 fl oz (150 ml) low-fat natural yogurt

1. Place the chicken in a non-metallic bowl and add the vinegar and salt. Stir well, cover and refrigerate for 30 minutes.
2. Mix together the remaining ingredients. Drain the chicken, discarding the vinegar. Add the yogurt marinade, stirring well, and then cover and refrigerate for at least 3–4 hours, or overnight if preferred.
3. Preheat the grill. Thread the chicken on to 6 skewers and grill for about 12–15 minutes, turning frequently, until golden brown.

Points per serving: 3
Total Points per recipe: 18

Cook's note:
Don't leave the chicken in the vinegar mixture for more than 30 minutes.

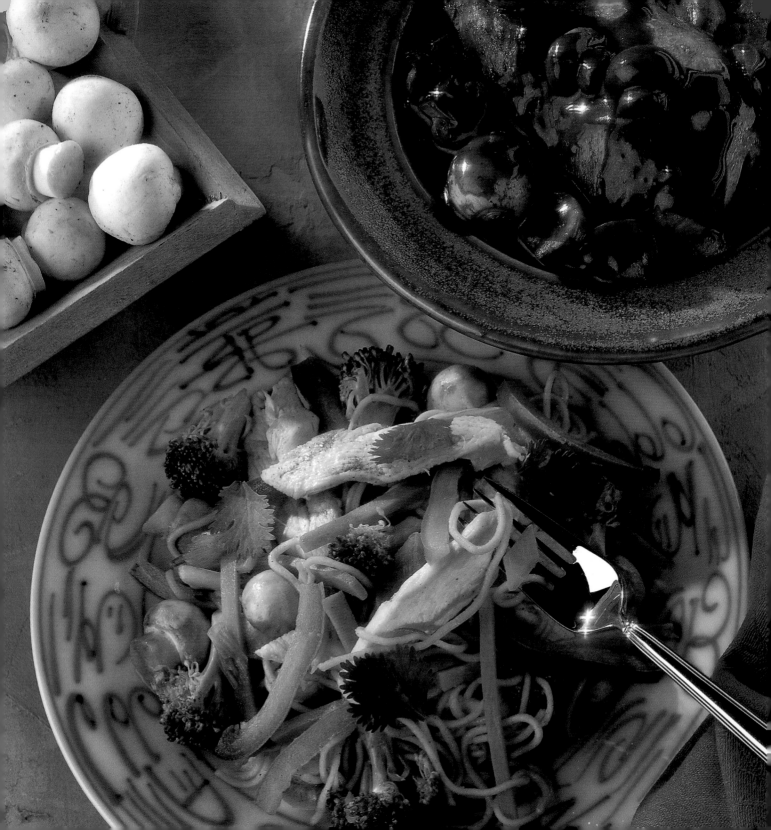

Chicken Stir-fry

Serves 4

Preparation time: 15 minutes
Cooking time: 10–12 minutes
Calories per serving: 350

Freezing: not recommended

V

Quick, colourful and very
nutritious, this simple stir-fry
tastes superb.

6 oz (180 g) Chinese thread egg
  noodles
1 tablespoon sesame or
  vegetable oil
a bunch of spring onions,
  trimmed and sliced

1 green or red pepper, de-seeded
  and sliced finely
1 large carrot, cut in thin strips
4 oz (120 g) broccoli florets
12 oz (360 g) skinless, boneless
  chicken, sliced in strips
8 oz (240 g) button mushrooms
1 teaspoon finely grated fresh
  root ginger
1 teaspoon Chinese five-spice
  powder
1 tablespoon chopped fresh
  coriander or parsley
1 tablespoon light soy sauce
salt and freshly ground black
  pepper
fresh coriander or parsley,
  to garnish

1. Soak the noodles in boiling water for 6 minutes, or according
to pack instructions.
2. Meanwhile, heat the oil in a wok or large frying-pan. Add the
spring onions, pepper, carrot, broccoli and chicken. Stir-fry over
a high heat for 5–6 minutes, until the chicken is cooked through.
The vegetables should remain crisp, crunchy and colourful.
3. Drain the noodles thoroughly. Add them to the wok with the
mushrooms, and stir-fry for 2 minutes. Add the ginger, five-spice
powder and coriander or parsley. Stir-fry for 1–2 minutes more
to heat thoroughly.
4. Season the stir-fry with the soy sauce, salt and pepper. Serve
on warm plates, garnished with fresh coriander or parsley.

Points per serving: 5
Total Points per recipe: 20

Variation:
Omit the noodles and serve the stir-fry with 6 oz (180 g) long-grain
rice, cooked according to pack instructions.

V Vegetarian option:
Substitute 8 oz (240 g) of smoked tofu for the chicken. This will
reduce the Points per serving to 4 and the Total Points per recipe
to 16.

Coq au Vin

Serves 4

Preparation time: 15 minutes
Cooking time: 40 minutes
Calories per serving: 220

Freezing: recommended

Lean chicken in a red wine
sauce with mushrooms and
shallots makes a perfect meal
for a special occasion.

1 tablespoon olive or
  vegetable oil

8 shallots or small onions,
  halved
1–2 garlic cloves, crushed
4 × 4 oz (120 g) skinless,
  boneless chicken breasts
4 fl oz (120 ml) red wine
1/2 pint (300 ml) chicken stock
6 oz (180 g) button
  mushrooms, halved
1 bay leaf (optional)
1 tablespoon cornflour, blended
  with 2 tablespoons cold water
salt and freshly ground black
  pepper

1. Heat the oil in a large frying pan or saucepan and sauté the
shallots or onions and garlic for about 5 minutes, until they begin
to turn brown. Remove them from the pan and set aside.
2. Add the chicken breasts to the pan and seal them quickly on
each side. Add the wine to the pan and bring it to the boil, allowing
it to bubble for a few seconds. Pour the chicken stock into the pan.
3. Return the shallots and garlic to the pan and add the
mushrooms and bay leaf (if using). Cover and simmer gently for
about 30 minutes, until the chicken is tender.
4. Stir the cornflour mixture into the pan juices. Heat, stirring
until thickened and smooth. Cook gently for 1 minute. Check
the seasoning, remove the bay leaf and serve.

Points per serving: 3.5
Total Points per recipe: 14

Chicken Pie

Serves 4

Preparation time: 25 minutes
Cooking time: 45 minutes
Calories per serving: 375

Freezing: recommended

Chicken, ham and sweetcorn, topped with sliced cooked potatoes, makes a satisfying main-course dish.

1½ lb (720 g) potatoes
4 teaspoons margarine
2 oz (60 g) plain white flour
½ pint (300 ml) skimmed milk
+ 2 tablespoons

½ pint (300 ml) chicken stock
8 oz (240 g) cooked chicken, cut in chunks
3 oz (90 g) cooked ham, chopped
3 oz (90 g) canned or frozen sweetcorn
2 teaspoons chopped fresh parsley or 1 teaspoon dried
1 egg
salt and freshly ground black pepper
chopped fresh parsley, to garnish

1. Cook the potatoes in plenty of lightly salted boiling water for about 15 minutes, until just tender. Drain and cool.
2. Preheat the oven to Gas Mark 6/200°C/400°F.
3. Meanwhile, melt 3 teaspoons of the margarine in a medium-sized saucepan. Add the flour, stirring to blend, and cook gently for 1 minute. Gradually add ½ pint (300 ml) skimmed milk, and then stir in the chicken stock. Heat, stirring constantly, until the sauce boils and thickens.

4. Add the chicken, ham, sweetcorn and parsley to the sauce. Season with salt and pepper.
5. Grease a shallow ovenproof dish with the remaining teaspoon of margarine. Pour in the chicken and ham mixture. Slice the cooked potatoes and arrange them over the top. Beat the egg and remaining 2 tablespoons of milk together and brush over the surface of the potatoes to glaze them.
6. Bake for 25–30 minutes, or until the potatoes are golden brown. Sprinkle with a little chopped fresh parsley and serve.

Points per serving: 7
Total Points per recipe: 28

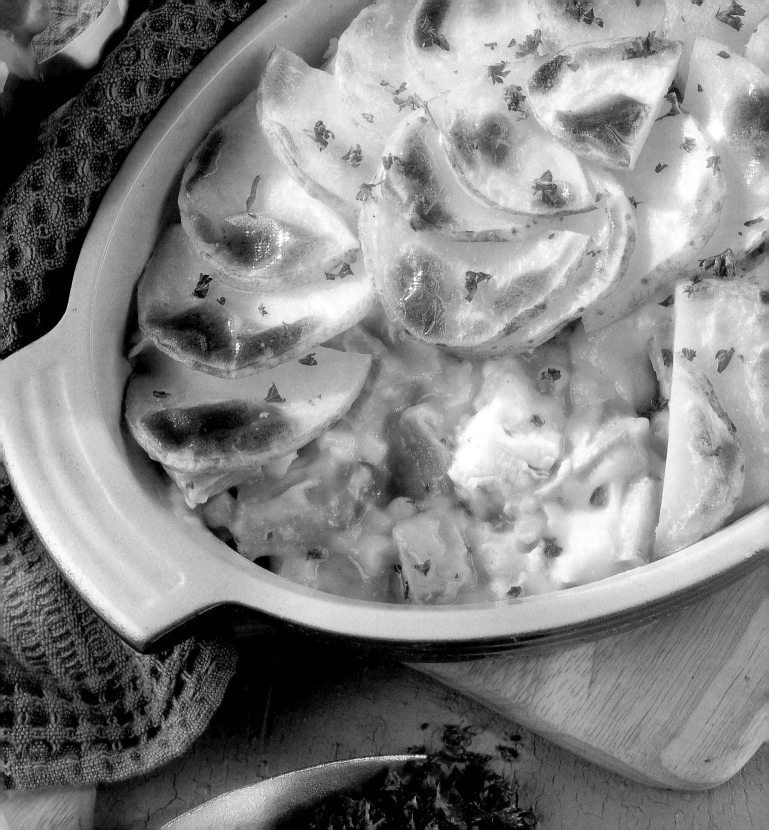

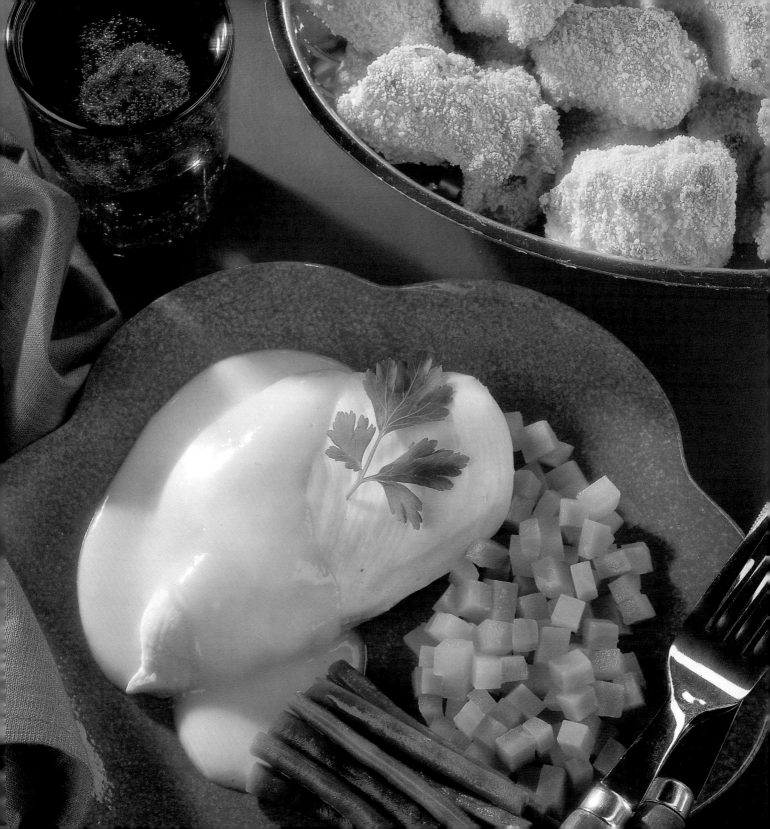

Chicken Supreme

Serves 4

Preparation time: 10 minutes
Cooking time: 25 minutes
Calories per serving: 270

Freezing: recommended

In this easy recipe, chicken breasts are gently poached, and then served with the cooking liquor, which is made into a sauce.

4 × 5 oz (150 g) skinless, boneless, chicken breasts
1 small onion, halved
1 bay leaf
1/2 chicken stock cube, dissolved in 1/2 pint (300 ml) boiling water
1/4 pint (150 ml) skimmed milk
1 oz (30 g) plain white flour
1 tablespoon margarine
salt and freshly ground black pepper
sprigs of fresh parsley, to garnish

1. Place the chicken breasts in a frying pan with the onion and bay leaf. Add the hot chicken stock, bring to the boil, and then reduce the heat and simmer gently for 20 minutes, turning the chicken over half-way through. Discard the onion and bay leaf.
2. Remove the chicken from the frying pan and keep warm. Strain 1/4 pint (150 ml) of the chicken stock into a small saucepan. Add the milk, flour and margarine, whisking to blend. Heat gently, stirring constantly with a small wire whisk, until blended and thickened. Cook gently for 1 minute. Season with salt and pepper to taste.
3. Serve the chicken on warmed plates, with steamed fresh vegetables. Pour an equal quantity of sauce over each chicken portion and serve at once, garnished with sprigs of fresh parsley.

Points per serving: 4
Total Points per recipe: 16

Chicken Nuggets

Serves 4

Preparation time: 10 minutes
Cooking time: 20 minutes
Calories per serving: 230

Freezing: recommended

Leaner – and more succulent – than shop-bought varieties, these chicken nuggets are very tasty.

2 tablespoons plain white flour, seasoned
15 oz (450 g) skinless, boneless chicken, cut in large chunks
1 egg
2 oz (60 g) dried breadcrumbs
1/2 teaspoon vegetable oil
salt and freshly ground black pepper

1. Preheat the oven to Gas Mark 5/190°C/375°F.
2. Sprinkle the seasoned flour on a plate and roll the pieces of chicken in it, to coat.
3. Beat the egg in a bowl with 2 tablespoons of cold water. Sprinkle the breadcrumbs on another plate. Grease a baking sheet with the oil.
4. Dip the floured chicken pieces into the egg, and then coat them with the breadcrumbs. Place them on the baking sheet and bake for approximately 20 minutes, or until crisp and golden brown.

Points per serving: 4
Total Points per recipe: 16

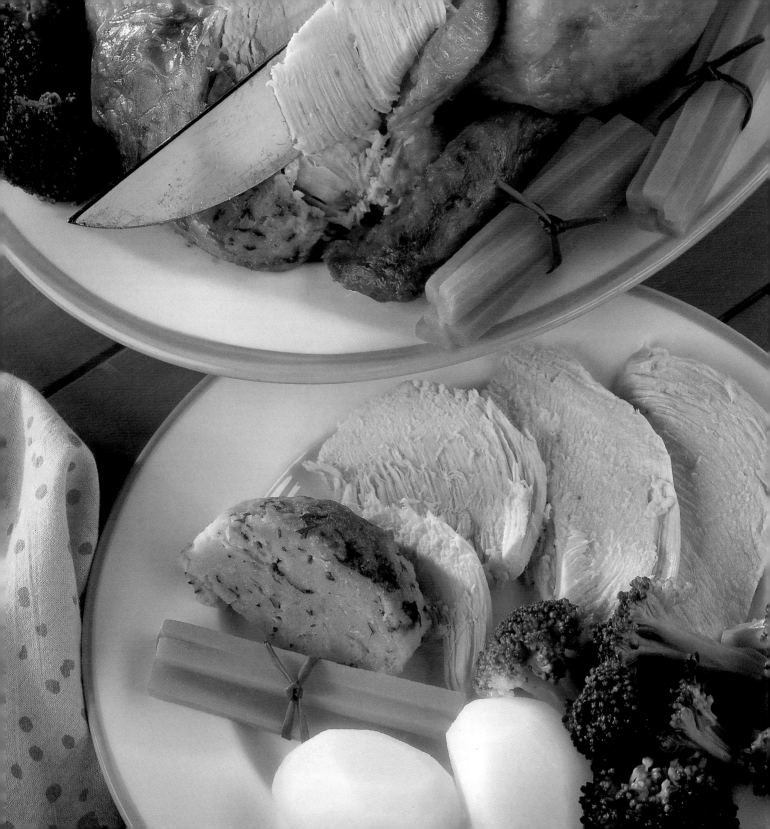

Roast Chicken

Serves 4

Preparation time: 10 minutes
Cooking time: 1 hour 25 minutes
Calories per serving: 235

Freezing: not recommended

The lemon zest and garlic in the stuffing give the chicken a fine flavour. If you're not keen on garlic, simply leave it out.

1 tablespoon vegetable oil
1 small onion, chopped finely
2 garlic cloves, crushed
1 egg
1 tablespoon chopped fresh chives or parsley
2 oz (60 g) fresh white or brown breadcrumbs
1 lemon
3 lb (1.5 kg) chicken, wiped
salt and freshly ground black pepper

1. Preheat the oven to Gas Mark 6/200°C/400°F.
2. Heat the oil in a small frying pan and sauté the onion and garlic for about 5 minutes, until softened.
3. Beat the egg in a mixing bowl and add the chives or parsley, breadcrumbs, onion and garlic. Finely grate the zest from the lemon and add to the stuffing mixture. Season with salt and pepper and stir well.
4. Cut the lemon in half and place it in the body cavity of the bird. (This gives the chicken a good flavour.) Loosely stuff the neck cavity with the breadcrumb stuffing.
5. Put the chicken in a roasting pan and cook for 1 hour 20 minutes (i.e. 20 minutes per 1 lb (480 g) of bird plus 20 minutes extra). Check that the bird is cooked by piercing the thickest part of the thigh with a sharp knife or skewer – the juices should run clear, not pink.
6. Carve the chicken, first removing any skin. Allow 4 oz (120 g) cooked chicken per person. Divide the stuffing equally between each portion and serve at once.

Points per serving: 5.5
Total Points per recipe: 22

Meat

The recipes in this chapter will show you the way forward to healthier meat-based meals. Beef, lamb, pork, liver and sausage recipes can all be found within these next few pages, from simple choices like Pork Chops with Apple Sauce (page 45) and Beefburgers (page 36), to new classics like Moussaka (page 43) and Chilli con Carne (page 40). These are all such delicious, comforting meals, it's no wonder they turn up so often on our supper tables! The advantage of the recipes here is that they have been trimmed down to make them healthier and kinder on the waistline. Even Toad-in-the-Hole (page 38) can make an appearance on the Programme once it has had the Weight Watchers treatment!

Sausage Casserole

Serves 4

Preparation time: 20 minutes
Cooking time: 1¼ hours
Calories per serving: 310

Freezing: recommended

12 oz (360 g) thin-link pork
  and beef sausages
2 teaspoons oil
1 large onion, sliced
1 large carrot, sliced
2 celery sticks, sliced

1 tablespoon paprika
1 teaspoon ground cumin
  (optional)
14 oz (420 g) canned chopped
  tomatoes
12 oz (360 g) canned mixed
  pulses, rinsed and drained
½ pint (300 ml) chicken stock
1 tablespoon cornflour, blended
  with 2 tablespoons cold water
salt and freshly ground
  black pepper

1. Preheat the oven to Gas Mark 5/190°C/375°F.
2. Preheat the grill. Place the sausages on the grill rack and grill for a few minutes, turning frequently, until the fat stops dripping and they're brown all over. Cut each sausage in half.
3. Heat the oil in a large flameproof casserole dish and sauté the onion for 3 minutes, until softened. Add the carrot and celery and cook for 3 minutes more, stirring frequently.
4. Add the paprika and cumin (if using), and then stir in the tomatoes and mixed pulses. Pour in the stock, and season with salt and pepper. Add the grilled sausages and stir gently.
5. Bake for 1 hour. Stir the cornflour mixture into the casserole. Cook for 5 minutes more, and then serve with fresh vegetables.

Points per serving: 7.5
Total Points per recipe: 30

Beefburgers

Serves 4

Preparation and cooking time:
20 minutes
Calories per serving: 370

Freezing: recommended

V

These home-made beefburgers taste much better than bought ones, and you will know exactly what goes into them.

12 oz (360 g) extra-lean
  minced beef

1 small onion, chopped very
  finely
1 tablespoon chopped fresh
  parsley or 1 teaspoon dried
a few drops of mushroom
  ketchup or Worcestershire
  sauce
1 small egg, beaten
salt and freshly ground
  black pepper
To serve:
4 × 2 oz (60 g) burger buns
  shredded lettuce
2 tomatoes, sliced

1. Combine the burger ingredients together in a large mixing bowl, or use a food processor or blender to mix the ingredients thoroughly.
2. Shape the mixture into 4 burgers. Wrap in clingfilm and refrigerate until needed.
3. Preheat the grill. Place the burgers on the grill rack and cook for about 5 minutes on each side, until the fat stops dripping.
4. Serve on burger buns, with plenty of shredded lettuce and sliced tomato.

Points per serving: 4.5
Total Points per recipe: 18

V Vegetarian option:
Substitute 8 oz (240 g) reconstituted soya mince for the minced beef. This will reduce the Points per serving to 3.5 and the Total Points per recipe to 14.

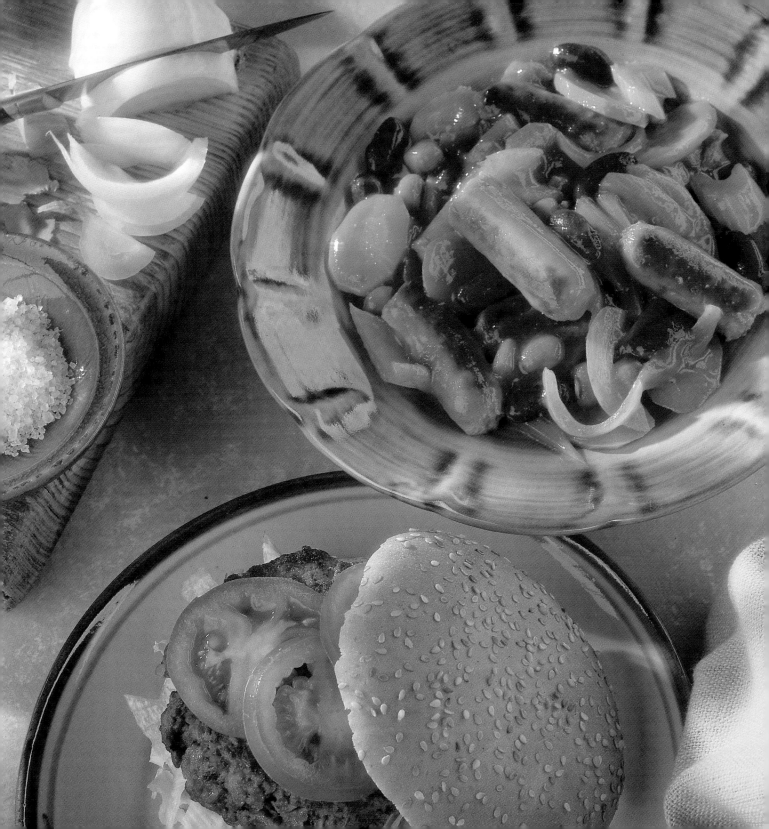

Toad-in-the-Hole

Serves 4

Preparation time: 20 minutes
Cooking time: 40 minutes
Calories per serving: 350

Freezing: not recommended

V

4 oz (120 g) plain white flour
½ teaspoon salt
1 egg
½ pint (300 ml) skimmed milk
12 oz (360 g) thin-link pork
  and beef sausages
2 tablespoons vegetable oil

A light and crispy batter is the secret of a successful toad-in-the-hole. Make sure that the oven has preheated properly, and avoid opening the oven door during cooking, or your batter may deflate!

1. Beat together the flour, salt, egg and milk in a large bowl, using a wire whisk or hand-held electric beater. Allow to stand for 10–15 minutes.
2. Preheat the grill. Place the sausages on the grill rack and cook, turning frequently, for about 10 minutes, or until the fat stops dripping.
3. Preheat the oven to Gas Mark 7/210°C/425°F. Heat the oil in a non-stick roasting pan until very hot.

4. Put the sausages into the roasting pan and pour the batter over. Return to the oven as quickly as possible and cook for 25–30 minutes, or until puffy and golden brown.

Points per serving: 9
Total Points per recipe: 36

V Vegetarian option:
Use vegetarian sausages, grilled very lightly. This will reduce the Points per serving to 7 and the Total Points per recipe to 28.

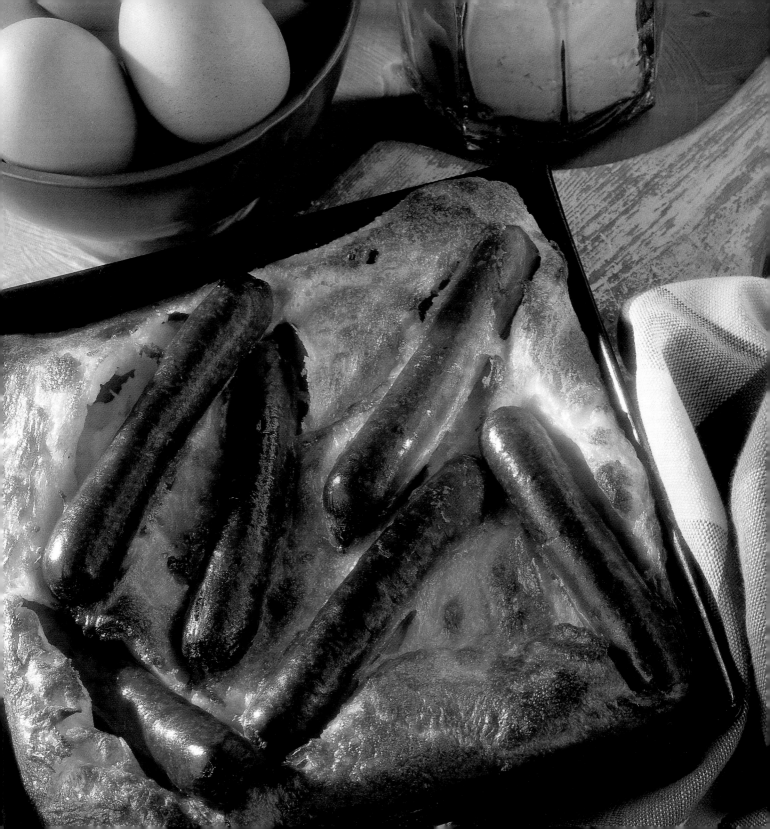

Goulash

Serves 4

Preparation time: 20 minutes
Cooking time: 1½ hours
Calories per serving: 245

Freezing: recommended

**This rich, warming stew
tastes all the better for its
long, slow cooking. Serve it
with creamed potatoes or rice.**

2 teaspoons vegetable oil
12 oz (360 g) lean stewing steak,
   cut in 1-inch (2.5 cm) cubes
1 large onion, sliced
1 garlic clove, crushed
2 tablespoons paprika
14 oz (420 g) canned chopped
   tomatoes
1 tablespoon tomato purée
1 large red pepper, de-seeded
   and chopped
1 beef stock cube, dissolved in
   ½ pint (300 ml) hot water
1 tablespoon cornflour, blended
   with 2 tablespoons cold water
salt and freshly ground black
   pepper
4 tablespoons low-fat natural
   yogurt, to serve
chopped fresh parsley,
   to garnish

1. Heat the oil in a large saucepan and add the steak, stirring it
round until sealed all over. Add the onion and garlic and sauté for
3–5 minutes, until softened. Add the paprika, stirring well.
2. Add the tomatoes, tomato purée, red pepper and stock to the
saucepan. Bring to the boil and then reduce the heat. Cover and
simmer for 1½ hours, until the meat is very tender. Check the level
of liquid from time to time, topping up with a little extra water if
necessary.
3. Season the goulash with salt and pepper. Add the blended
cornflour and stir until thickened. Cook for 1 minute. Serve,
topped with one tablespoon of yogurt per portion, and garnished
with parsley.

Points per serving: 4
Total Points per recipe: 16

Chilli con Carne

Serves 4

Preparation time: 15 minutes
Cooking time: 40 minutes
Calories per serving: 415

Freezing: recommended

V

**Extra vegetables and less meat
make a very tasty chilli, with
less fat and fewer Calories,
but just as much flavour.**

12 oz (360 g) extra-lean
   minced beef
1 large onion, chopped
2 garlic cloves, chopped
2 celery sticks, sliced
1 red or green pepper, de-seeded
   and chopped
2–3 teaspoons medium-
   strength chilli powder
14 oz (420 g) canned chopped
   tomatoes
1 tablespoon tomato purée
12 oz (360 g) canned red kidney
   beans, rinsed and drained
¼ pint (150 ml) vegetable stock
6 oz (180 g) long-grain rice
salt and freshly ground black
   pepper

1. Dry-fry the minced beef in a large non-stick saucepan until
browned, stirring all the time to break it up. Add the onion and
garlic and sauté for about 5 minutes, stirring often.
2. Add the celery, pepper, chilli powder, tomatoes, tomato purée, red
kidney beans and stock. Bring to the boil, and then cover and reduce
the heat. Simmer for about 30 minutes, stirring occasionally.
3. Meanwhile, about 15 minutes before the chilli is cooked,
boil the rice in plenty of lightly salted boiling water for about
12 minutes, until tender. Drain well and rinse with boiling water.
4. Season the chilli according to taste. Divide the cooked rice
between 4 warm serving plates and pile the chilli on top. Serve
at once.

Points per serving: 6
Total Points per recipe: 24

V Vegetarian option:
Replace the minced beef with 10 oz (300 g) of reconstituted soya
mince. This will reduce the Points per serving to 5 and the Total
Points per recipe to 20.

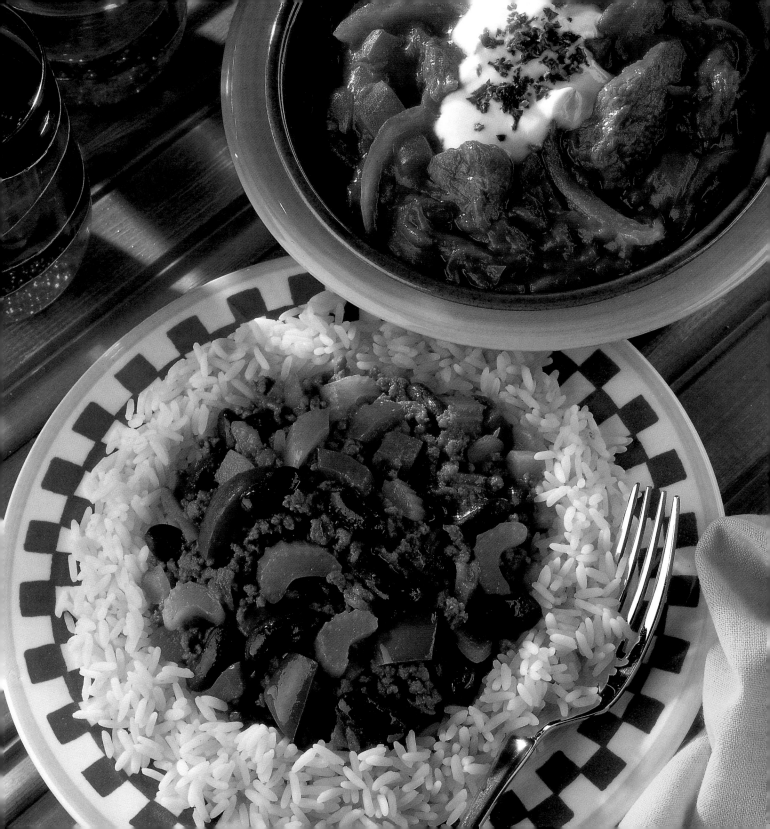

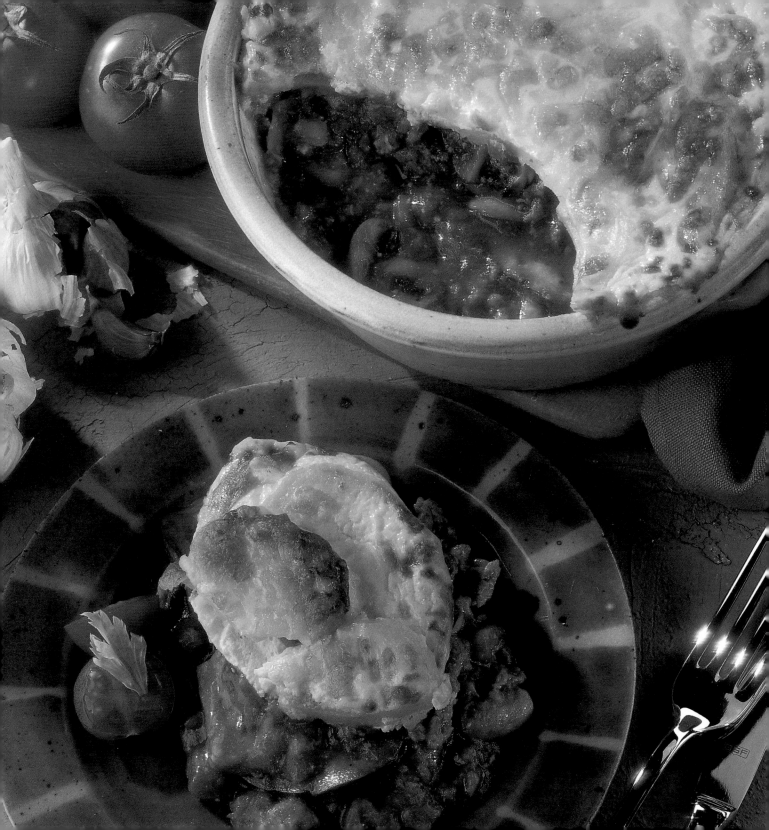

Moussaka

Serves 4

Preparation time: 25 minutes
Cooking time: 1 hour
10 minutes
Calories per serving: 380

Freezing: recommended

Use minced lamb or beef to
make this delicious moussaka.
Either way, choose very lean
meat to keep the Calories
to a minimum.

1 large aubergine, sliced
12 oz (360 g) extra-lean minced
  lamb or beef
1 onion, chopped finely
1 garlic clove, crushed
8 oz (240 g) mushrooms, wiped
  and sliced
14 oz (420 g) canned chopped
  tomatoes
1/4 pint (150 ml) lamb or beef
  stock
2 tablespoons cornflour,
  blended with 4 tablespoons
  cold water
1 lb (480 g) potatoes, par-boiled
  and sliced
1 egg
5 fl oz (150 ml) low-fat natural
  yogurt
1 oz (30 g) Cheddar cheese,
  grated
salt and freshly ground
  black pepper

1. Sprinkle the aubergine slices with salt, leave for 10 minutes,
and then turn the slices over and repeat. Place them in a colander,
rinse and drain well.
2. Dry-fry the mince until browned, stirring all the time to break
it up. Add the onion and garlic and sauté for 3–4 minutes. Add the
mushrooms and cook for 5 minutes more. Stir in the tomatoes
and stock, bring to the boil, and then simmer for 10 minutes.
3. Stir the blended cornflour into the saucepan and cook, stirring
constantly, until thickened.

4. Preheat the oven to Gas Mark 5/190°C/375°F.
5. Spoon half the mince mixture into an ovenproof baking dish.
Layer the aubergine slices over the top. Spread with the remaining
mince mixture and then arrange the sliced potatoes in an
overlapping layer on top.
6. Beat together the egg and yogurt. Season well and pour over the
potatoes to cover them completely. Sprinkle with the grated cheese
and bake for 45 minutes, until the topping is set and golden brown.

Points per serving: 5.5
Total Points per recipe: 22

Cook's note:
Salting and draining the aubergine extracts any bitter juices which
may interfere with the flavour of the dish.

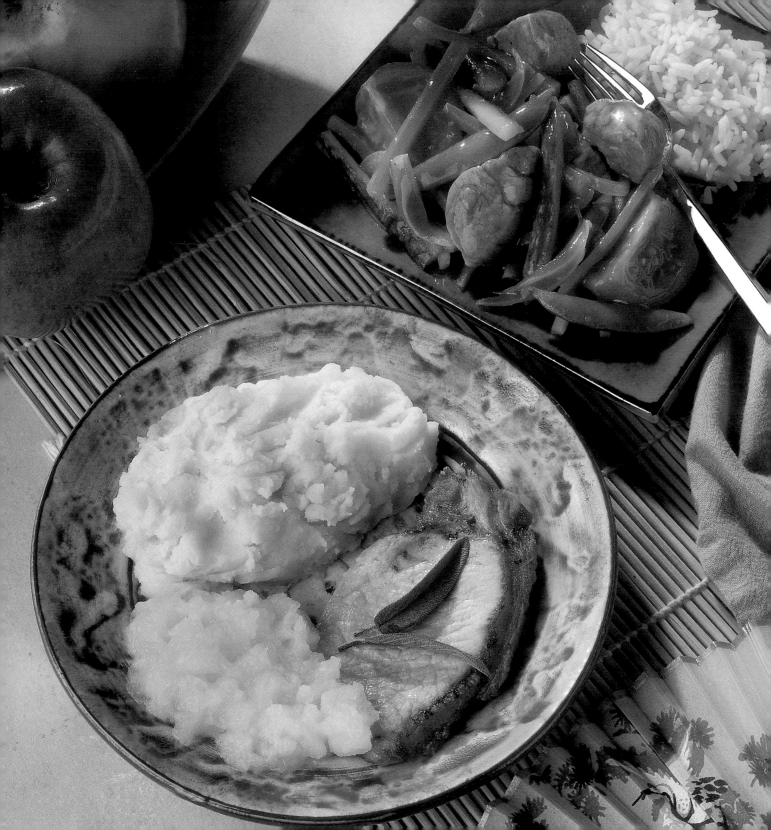

Sweet and Sour Pork

Serves 4

Preparation time: 15 minutes
Cooking time: 40 minutes
Calories per serving: 305

Freezing: recommended

Lean shoulder or leg of pork
are ideal cuts to use for
this dish.

2 teaspoons vegetable oil
10 oz (300 g) lean pork, cut in
  cubes
1 garlic clove, crushed
1 onion, sliced
1 small carrot, cut in
  matchsticks
3 oz (90 g) sugar snap peas or
  green beans
½ pint (300 ml) vegetable stock
3-inch (7.5 cm) piece of
  cucumber, sliced in
  matchsticks
3 tomatoes, skinned and
  quartered
4 oz (120 g) long-grain rice
1 tablespoon cornflour
1 tablespoon caster sugar
2 tablespoons vinegar
2 tablespoons light soy sauce
salt and freshly ground
  black pepper

1. Heat the oil in a large frying pan and brown the pork all over.
Add the garlic and sauté for 2 minutes. Add the onion, carrot and
sugar snap peas or green beans, and then pour in the stock. Bring
to the boil, and then reduce the heat and simmer gently for 20–30
minutes, until the pork is tender. Add the cucumber and tomatoes.
2. Meanwhile, cook the rice in plenty of lightly salted boiling water
for about 12 minutes, until tender.
3. Blend the cornflour, sugar, vinegar and soy sauce. Stir this into
the pork and vegetable mixture and cook for 2–3 minutes, until
thickened. Season to taste.
4. Serve on warm plates with the drained, cooked rice.

Points per serving: 4.5
Total Points per recipe: 18

Pork Chops with Apple Sauce

Serves 4

Preparation and cooking time:
20 minutes
Calories per serving: 385

Freezing: not recommended

Well-grilled pork chops with
a tart apple sauce and creamy
mashed potatoes make a
welcome mid-week meal.

2 lb (960 g) potatoes, peeled
  and quartered
½ teaspoon salt
4 × 5 oz (150 g) pork chops,
  trimmed
a few sprigs of fresh sage
  (optional)
1 lb (480 g) cooking apples,
  peeled, cored and chopped
3 tablespoons water
4 tablespoons skimmed milk

1. Put the potatoes in a large saucepan and cover with cold water.
Add the salt, bring to the boil, and then cover and reduce the heat.
Cook for about 20 minutes, or until the potatoes are tender.
2. Meanwhile, preheat the grill. Place the pork chops on the grill
rack and top each with a sprig of sage (if using). Grill them for
about 10 minutes on each side.
3. Put the apples in a saucepan with the water and cook them over
a low heat until soft. Beat them with a wooden spoon until pulpy.
4. Mash the potatoes and add the milk, beating well until smooth
and creamy.
5. Serve the pork chops with the mashed potatoes and apple sauce.

Points per serving: 9.5
Total Points per recipe: 38

Beef Stew and Dumplings

Serves 4

Preparation time: 25 minutes
Cooking time: 2 hours
10 minutes
Calories per serving: 220

Freezing: recommended

**The ultimate comfort food –
just the thing for a cold
winter's day.**

1 tablespoon vegetable oil
1 lb (480 g) braising steak,
   cubed
8 shallots or small onions,
   halved
2 celery sticks, chopped
1 large carrot, sliced
1 turnip, chopped
1 tablespoon plain white flour
1 beef stock cube, dissolved in
   $^3/_4$ pint (450 ml) boiling
   water
$^1/_2$ teaspoon dried mixed herbs
salt and freshly ground
   black pepper
For the dumplings:
3 oz (90 g) self-raising flour
a pinch of salt
$^1/_2$ teaspoon dried mixed herbs
2 tablespoons margarine

1. Preheat the oven to Gas Mark 3/170°C/325°F.
2. Heat the oil in a flameproof casserole and brown the steak all
over. Add the shallots or onions, celery, carrot and turnip, and cook
for about 5 minutes, stirring occasionally. Remove from the heat
and stir in the flour. Add the stock and herbs. Season with salt and
pepper, transfer to the oven and cook for 1$^1/_2$ hours.
3. To make the dumplings, sift the flour and salt into a bowl. Mix
in the dried herbs, and then rub in the margarine until the mixture
resembles fine breadcrumbs. Add just enough cold water to make
a soft, but not sticky dough. Shape 8 small dumplings and add
them to the casserole. Cover and cook for 30 minutes more,
or until the meat is tender.
4. Serve the casserole with two dumplings per portion.

Points per serving: 7
Total Points per recipe: 28

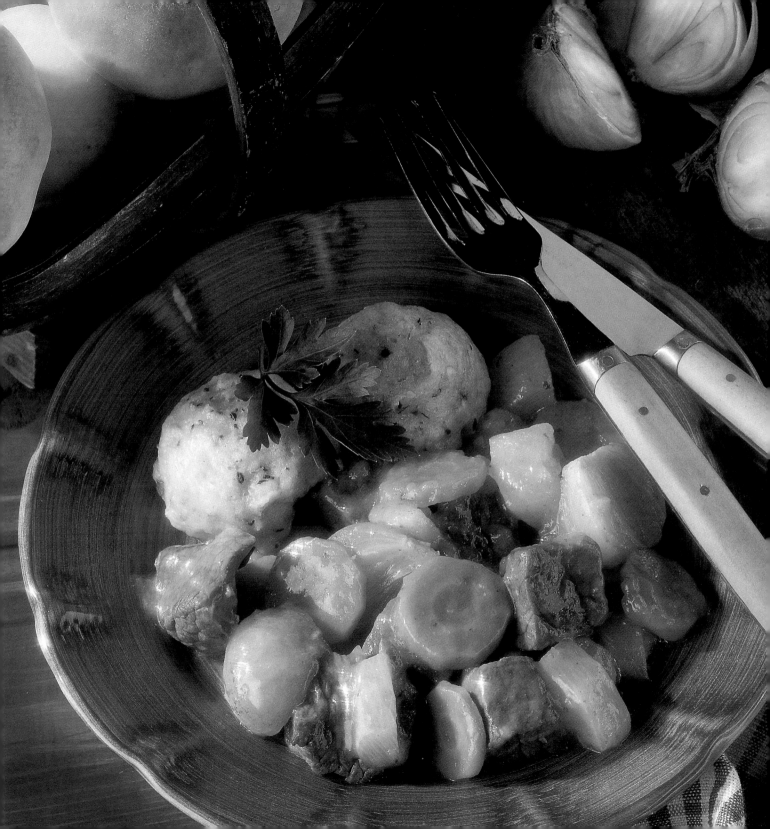

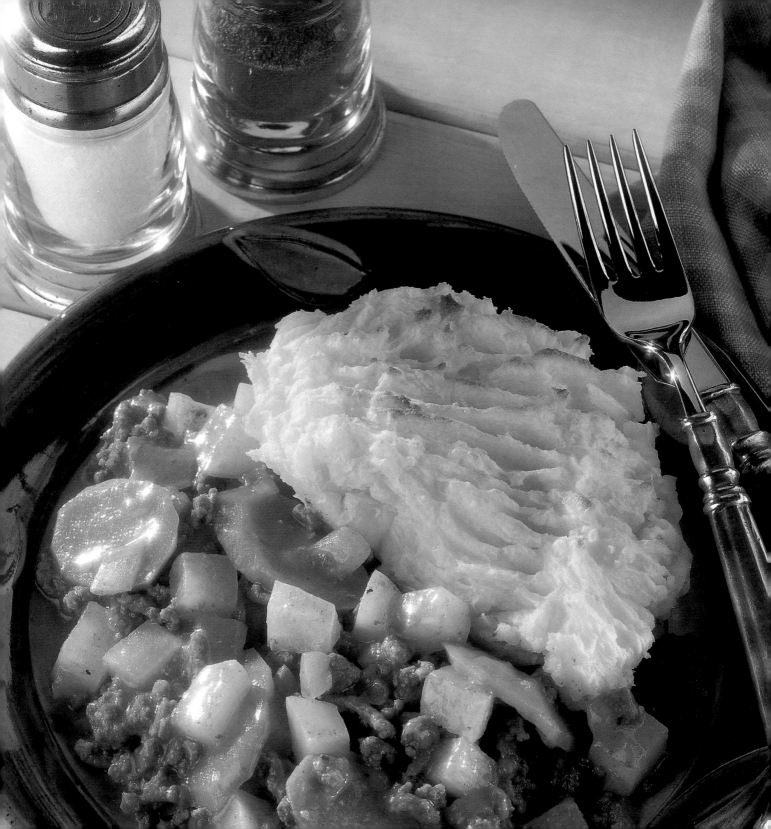

Cottage Pie

Serves 4

Preparation time: 20 minutes
Cooking time: 1 hour
Calories per serving: 405

Freezing: recommended

V

Extra vegetables add padding to this traditional favourite, without adding any to you!

2 lb (960 g) potatoes, peeled and quartered
$^1/_2$ teaspoon salt
12 oz (360 g) extra-lean minced beef
1 large onion, chopped finely
2 carrots, sliced
1 turnip, chopped
$^1/_2$ pint (300 ml) vegetable stock
4 tablespoons skimmed milk
1 tablespoon cornflour, blended with 2 tablespoons cold water
salt and freshly ground black pepper

1. Place the potatoes in a large saucepan and cover with cold water. Add the salt and bring to the boil. Cover and reduce the heat, and then simmer for about 20 minutes, until the potatoes are tender.
2. Meanwhile, dry-fry the minced beef in a large non-stick saucepan until browned, stirring all the time to break it up. Add the onion and sauté for about 3 minutes. Add the carrots and turnip, and then pour in the stock. Bring to the boil, and then cover and simmer for about 20 minutes.
3. Drain the potatoes and mash well. Add the milk and seasoning, and then beat vigorously with a wooden spoon or use a hand-held electric beater to whisk the potatoes until light and fluffy.

4. Add the blended cornflour to the beef mixture, stirring until thickened. Remove from the heat.
5. Preheat the oven to Gas Mark 5/190°C/375°F.
6. Transfer the meat mixture to an ovenproof dish and top with the mashed potato. Bake for 25–30 minutes, until heated through and golden brown on top.

Points per serving: 5
Total Points per recipe: 20

V Vegetarian option:
Substitute 10 oz (300 g) reconstituted soya mince for the beef. This will reduce the Points per serving to 4 and the Total Points per recipe to 16.

Lancashire Hot-Pot

Serves 4

Preparation time: 15 minutes
Cooking time: 1 hour
Calories per serving: 410

Freezing: not recommended

This must be one of the tastiest ways to enjoy lean lamb cutlets.

1¹/₂ lb (720 g) potatoes, peeled and sliced

3 onions, sliced in rings
1 teaspoon chopped fresh thyme or a large pinch of dried
1 lamb or beef stock cube, dissolved in ³/₄ pint (450 ml) boiling water
8 × 3 oz (90 g) lean lamb cutlets, trimmed of visible fat
salt and freshly ground black pepper
sprigs of fresh thyme, to garnish

1. Preheat the oven to Gas Mark 5/190°C/375°F.
2. Layer the potatoes and onions in a 3-pint (2-litre) ovenproof dish, seasoning lightly between each layer, and ending with a layer of potatoes.
3. Add the thyme to the stock and pour over the potatoes. Cover and bake for about 45 minutes, or until tender.
4. When the potatoes have been cooking for 25 minutes, preheat the grill to medium-hot. Arrange the lamb cutlets on the grill rack. Season lightly and grill them until the fat stops dripping (about 10 minutes on each side).
5. Remove the baking dish from the oven and arrange the lamb cutlets on top of the potatoes. Return the dish to the oven for a further 10–15 minutes to brown the potatoes.
6. Serve, garnished with sprigs of thyme.

Points per serving: 9
Total Points per recipe: 36

Liver and Onions

Serves 4

Preparation time: 10 minutes
Cooking time: 20 minutes
Calories per serving: 285

Freezing: not recommended

An ideal dish for eating economically – liver and onions fit the bill perfectly!

1 lb (480 g) lamb's liver, trimmed and sliced thinly

2 tablespoons plain white flour, seasoned
1 teaspoon dried mixed herbs (optional)
1 tablespoon vegetable oil
2 onions, sliced in rings
1 lamb or chicken stock cube dissolved in ¹/₂ pint (300 ml) boiling water
salt and freshly ground black pepper

1. Rinse the liver and pat it dry with kitchen paper.
2. Sprinkle the seasoned flour on a plate and add the dried mixed herbs, if using. Toss the liver in the flour to coat it well.
3. Heat the oil in a frying pan and add the onions. Sauté for about 5 minutes, until softened.
4. Add the liver to the frying pan and cook for 1–2 minutes on each side. Avoid over-cooking the liver as it will become tough. Pour in the stock and bring to the boil, stirring constantly. Reduce the heat and simmer gently for about 10 minutes.
5. Serve the liver and onions with mashed potatoes and fresh vegetables, adding the necessary Points.

Points per serving: 4.5
Total Points per recipe: 18

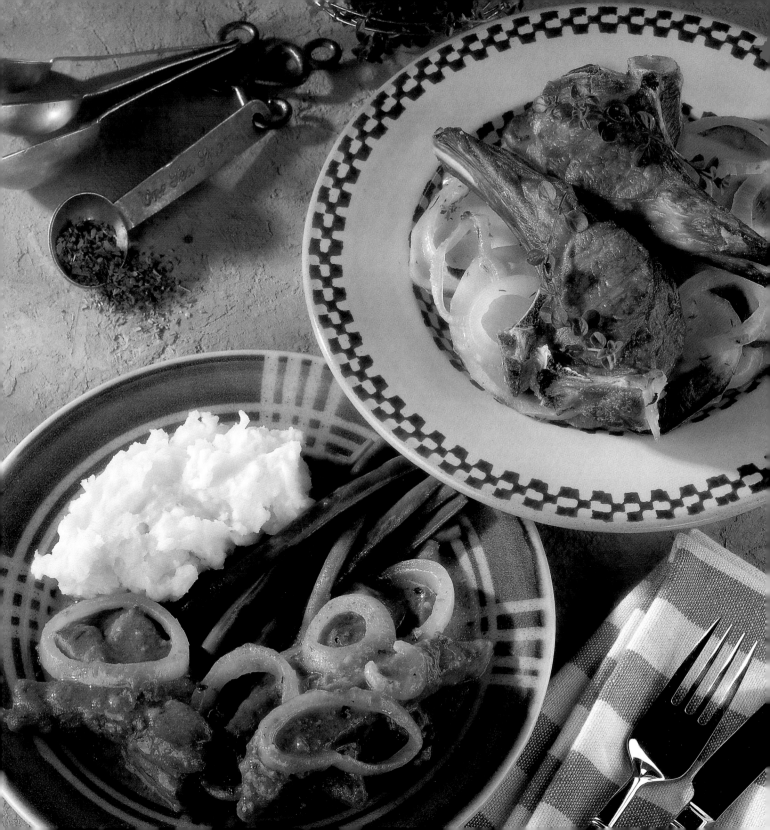

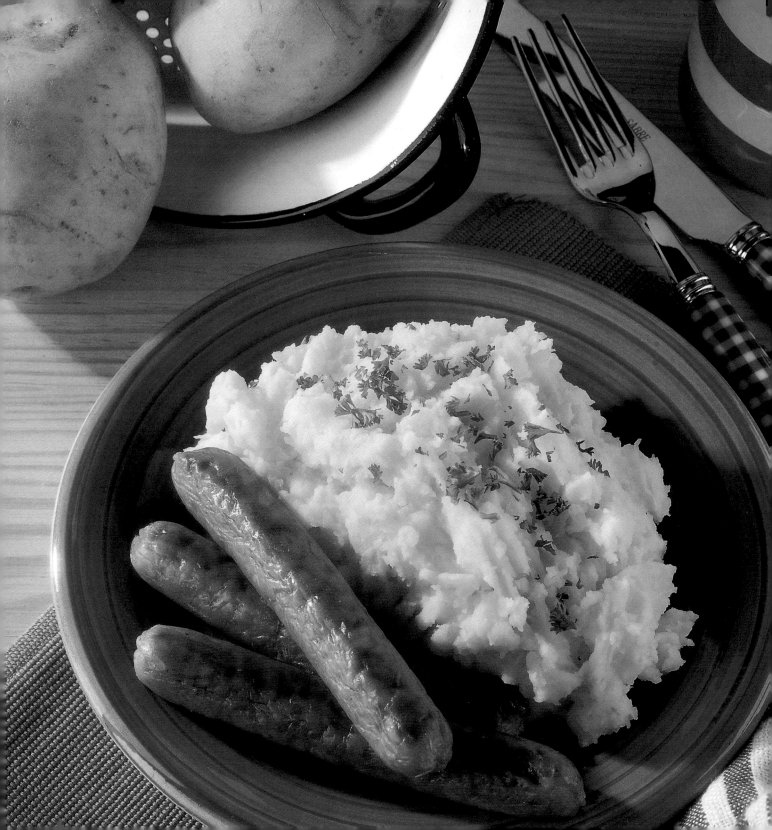

Sausage and Mash

Serves 4

Preparation time: 10 minutes
Cooking time: 25 minutes
Calories per serving: 305

Freezing: not recommended

V

Choose fat-reduced sausages to keep the Calories as low as possible.

2 lb (960 g) potatoes, peeled and quartered
1/2 teaspoon salt
12 oz (360 g) fat-reduced pork and beef sausages
4 tablespoons skimmed milk
salt and freshly ground black pepper

1. Place the potatoes in a large saucepan and cover with cold water. Add the salt and bring to the boil. Cover and reduce the heat, and then simmer for about 20 minutes, until the potatoes are tender.
2. Meanwhile, grill the sausages, turning them frequently, until the fat stops dripping and they are well browned.
3. Drain the potatoes and mash well. Add the milk and seasoning, and then beat vigorously with a wooden spoon to make the potatoes light and fluffy. Alternatively, use a hand-held electric beater to whisk the potatoes.

4. Reheat the potatoes over a low heat, stirring constantly to prevent them from burning on the base of the saucepan. Serve with the sausages.

Points per serving: 5.5
Total Points per recipe: 22

Weight Watchers note:
Prick the sausages with a fork before grilling. This will encourage as much fat as possible to escape during cooking.

V Vegetarian option:
Use 10 oz (300 g) vegetarian sausage, grilled according to pack instructions. Points per serving and Total Points per recipe will stay the same.

Vegetarian Meals

Whether or not you are vegetarian, you are bound to enjoy the recipes in this chapter. Nutritious, colourful and delicious, the Vegetable Chilli (page 60) is made with masses of fresh vegetables and red kidney beans for protein. Vegeburgers (see below) will prove that you can make a very tasty burger using soya mince, and the Bean and Lentil Stew (page 60) is the perfect recipe for warming you up on a cold winter's day. Serve any of these recipes as a welcome change from meat-based meals. They are economical, extremely tasty and a terrific introduction to vegetarian cooking – the Weight Watchers way.

Vegeburgers

Serves 4

Preparation time: 30 minutes
Cooking time: 10 minutes
Calories per serving: 285

Freezing: recommended

A clever combination of soya mince and seasonings makes these home-made vegetarian burgers just as tasty as the real thing.

3 oz (90 g) dehydrated soya mince

¼ pint (150 ml) vegetable stock
1 very small onion, chopped finely
2 oz (60 g) plain white flour
1 teaspoon dried mixed herbs
1 small egg, beaten
1 teaspoon mushroom ketchup or soy sauce
2 teaspoons vegetable oil
salt and freshly ground black pepper
4 × 2 oz (60 g) burger buns, to serve
lettuce, cucumber and tomato, to garnish

1. Place the soya mince in a bowl and pour the hot stock over. Allow to soak for about 10 minutes, or until the liquid is absorbed.
2. Preheat the grill.
3. Add the chopped onion, flour, herbs, egg and mushroom ketchup or soy sauce. Mix well and season with salt and pepper. Shape the mixture into 4 burgers.
4. Place the burgers on a grill pan and brush with a little vegetable oil. Grill for about 5 minutes and then turn over, brush with a little more oil and cook for 5 minutes more, or until browned.

5. Serve at once in the split burger buns, garnished with lettuce, cucumber and tomato.

Points per serving: 4.5
Total Points per recipe: 18

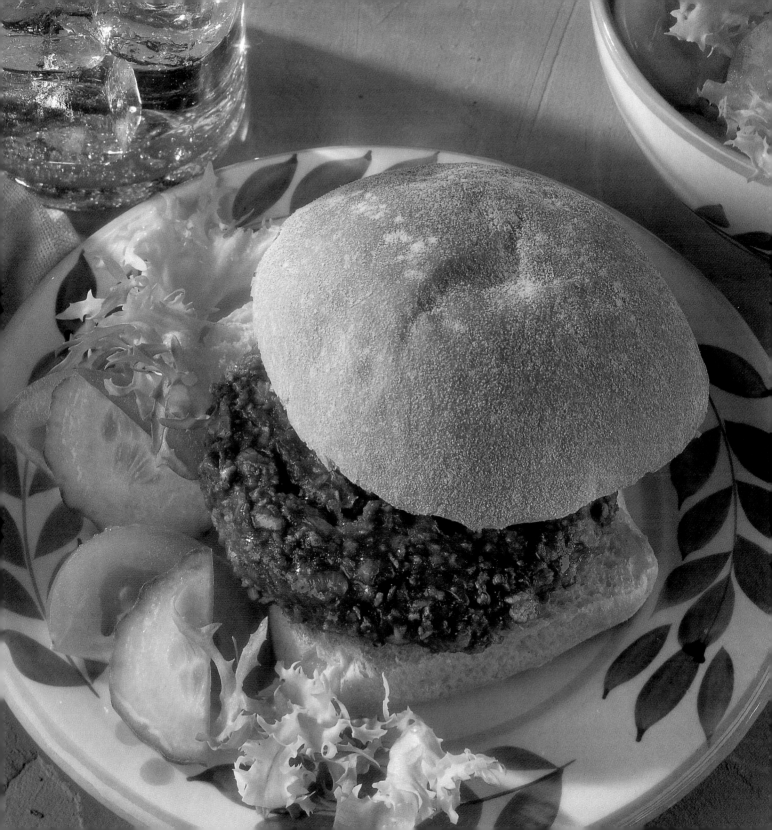

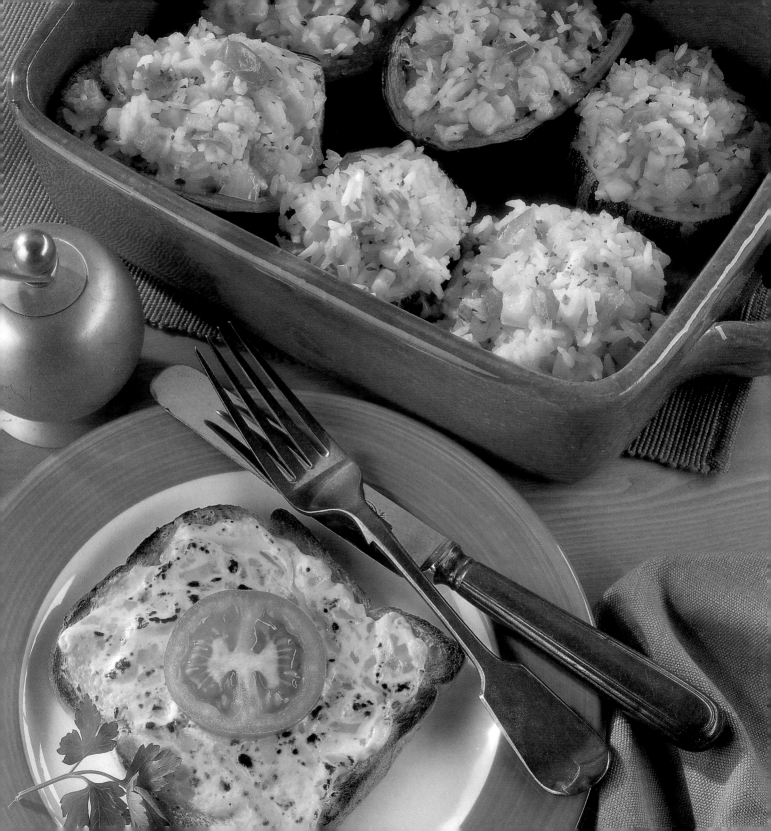

Stuffed Vegetables

Serves 4

Preparation time: 20 minutes
Cooking time: 30 minutes
Calories per serving: 410

Freezing: not recommended

Ⓥ If using vegetarian Cheddar

**Choose from a selection of
vegetables to pack with this
tasty filling, and then bake in
the oven for a nutritious and
delicious meat-free meal.**

1 tablespoon olive oil
1 onion, chopped finely
1 garlic clove, crushed
   (optional)
2 tomatoes, chopped
6 oz (180 g) cooked long-grain
   rice
6 oz (180 g) frozen sweetcorn
½ teaspoon dried mixed herbs
4 oz (120 g) mature Cheddar
   cheese, grated
vegetables of your choice, for
   stuffing (e.g. 1 marrow, 4 large
   courgettes, 2 large aubergines,
   8 large flat mushrooms,
   or 4 beef tomatoes)
salt and freshly ground
   black pepper

1. To make the filling, heat the olive oil in a small saucepan and
sauté the onion and garlic for about 4–5 minutes, or until softened.
2. Add the tomatoes and cook until pulpy, and then add the cooked
rice and sweetcorn. Stir in the herbs and cheese, and remove from
the heat. Season to taste with salt and pepper. Preheat the oven
to Gas Mark 5/190°C/375°F.
3. Prepare the vegetables for stuffing. If using marrow, slice it
thickly and scoop out the seeds and discard them. If using
courgettes, halve them lengthways, scoop out the seeds and discard
them. If using tomatoes, cut a slice off the tops, scoop out the seeds
and add them to the filling. If using aubergines, halve them and
scoop out the middle, and sprinkle each half liberally with salt,
leave for 10 minutes and then rinse and pat dry. If using
mushrooms, remove the stalks, chop them finely and add them
to the filling.
4. Arrange the prepared vegetables in a baking dish and pack them
with the filling. Cover and bake for 20–25 minutes, until cooked
and golden brown.

Points per serving: 7
Total Points per recipe: 28

Welsh Rarebit

Serves 4

Preparation time: 10 minutes
Cooking time: 10 minutes
Calories per serving: 175

Freezing: not recommended

Ⓥ If using vegetarian cheese

**Use a well-flavoured Cheddar
or Lancashire cheese to make
this tasty, but low-Calorie
rarebit.**

4 oz (120 g) low-fat soft cheese
2 oz (60 g) mature Cheddar
   or Lancashire cheese,
   grated finely
½ teaspoon Worcestershire
   sauce
¼ teaspoon mustard
4 × 1 oz (30 g) slices bread
freshly ground black pepper
tomato slices, to garnish

1. Combine the soft cheese, Cheddar or Lancashire cheese,
Worcestershire sauce and mustard in a small bowl. Season with
a little black pepper.
2. Lightly toast the bread on both sides. Spread the cheese mixture
on one side, and then grill until golden and bubbling.
3. Cut each toast in half and top with a slice of tomato. Serve
at once.

Points per serving: 3.5
Total Points per recipe: 14

Onion Quiche

Serves 4

Preparation time: 20 minutes
+ 15 minutes chilling
Cooking time: 50 minutes
Calories per serving: 360

Freezing: recommended

**Spanish onions are a good
choice for this delicious
savoury tart.**

2 teaspoons olive oil
2 large onions, sliced in rings

1 small red pepper, de-seeded
  and sliced
2 eggs
4 oz (120 g) low-fat soft cheese
8 tablespoons skimmed milk
1 tablespoon chopped fresh
  mixed herbs or 1 teaspoon
  dried mixed herbs
salt and freshly ground black
  pepper
For the pastry:
4 oz (120 g) plain white flour
a pinch of salt
4 tablespoons margarine,
  chilled
4 teaspoons cold water

1. To make the pastry, sift the flour and salt together in a large
bowl. Add the margarine and rub in, using your fingertips, until
the mixture resembles fine breadcrumbs.
2. Mix in the water, using a round-bladed knife, until the mixture
starts to form a ball. Draw together and knead lightly to form a
smooth dough, but avoid overhandling. Wrap in clingfilm and chill
for 15 minutes.
3. Preheat the oven to Gas Mark 6/200°C/400°F. Roll the dough
out thinly on a lightly floured surface, and line an 8-inch (20 cm)
flan dish. Place the flan dish on a baking sheet, line it with foil
or greaseproof paper and fill it with dried baking beans. Bake for
10 minutes, or until lightly browned.

4. Remove the lining and beans and allow the flan case to cool
slightly. Reduce the oven temperature to Gas Mark 4/180°C/350°F.
5. Meanwhile, heat the oil in a frying pan and sauté the onions
and pepper for about 5 minutes, until softened.
6. Arrange the onions and pepper in the flan case. Beat together the
eggs, soft cheese, milk and herbs. Season with salt and pepper and
pour over the onions and red pepper. Return to the oven and bake
for 25–30 minutes, or until set. Cool slightly before serving.

Points per serving: 6
Total Points per recipe: 24

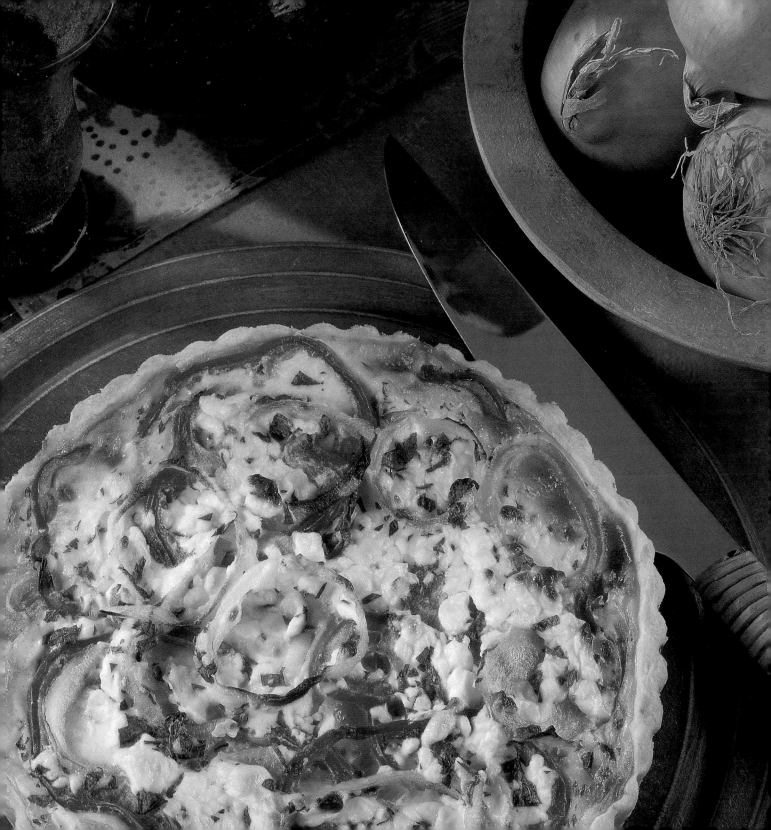

Bean and Lentil Stew

Serves 4

Preparation time: 20 minutes
Cooking time: 50 minutes
Calories per serving: 245

Freezing: recommended

A warming, comforting stew,
perfect for crisp autumn
evenings.

1 tablespoon margarine
1 large onion, chopped
1 garlic clove, crushed
1 carrot, sliced
2 celery sticks, sliced
1 tablespoon paprika
1 tablespoon chopped fresh
    coriander or parsley
14 oz (420 g) canned chopped
    tomatoes
15 oz (450 g) canned mixed
    pulses, rinsed and drained
1 oz (30 g) red lentils
¼ pint (150 ml) vegetable stock
6 oz (180 g) Quorn™ cubes
salt and freshly ground
    black pepper
chopped fresh coriander or
    parsley, to garnish

1. Melt the margarine in a large saucepan and sauté the onion
and garlic for about 5 minutes, until softened.
2. Add the carrot and celery and cook for 2 minutes more, and
then stir in the paprika and coriander or parsley.
3. Add the tomatoes, mixed pulses and lentils. Pour in the
vegetable stock. Bring to the boil, cover, and then reduce the heat
and simmer for 20 minutes, stirring occasionally.
4. Add the Quorn™ cubes to the saucepan and cook for 20 minutes
more, stirring occasionally. Season to taste.
5. Serve hot, garnished with chopped fresh coriander or parsley.

Points per serving: 4.5
Total Points per recipe: 18

Vegetable Chilli

Serves 4

Preparation time: 15 minutes
Cooking time: 35 minutes
Calories per serving: 305

Freezing: recommended

Lots of fresh vegetables and
spices make this a very
enjoyable vegetarian chilli.

1 tablespoon vegetable oil
1 large onion, chopped
1 large carrot, chopped
2 garlic cloves, chopped
1 large red or green pepper,
    de-seeded and chopped
8 oz (240 g) mushrooms, wiped
    and sliced
2 teaspoons mild or hot chilli
    powder
14 oz (420 g) canned chopped
    tomatoes
2 tablespoons tomato purée
14 oz (420 g) canned red kidney
    beans, rinsed and drained
½ pint (300 ml) vegetable stock
1 teaspoon dried mixed herbs
2 tablespoons cornflour,
    blended with 4 tablespoons
    cold water
salt and freshly ground
    black pepper
4 oz (120 g) long-grain rice,
    to serve

1. Heat the oil in a large saucepan and sauté the onion, carrot,
garlic and pepper for 3–4 minutes, until softened. Add the
mushrooms and chilli powder and cook for 2 minutes more.
2. Pour in the tomatoes and stir in the tomato purée. Add the
kidney beans, stock and herbs, and then bring to the boil. Reduce
the heat, cover and simmer for 20–30 minutes.
3. Meanwhile, cook the rice in plenty of lightly salted boiling
water for about 12 minutes, until tender. Drain and rinse with
boiling water.
4. Add the blended cornflour to the chilli, stirring until thickened.
Taste and adjust the seasoning with salt, pepper and a little extra
chilli powder, if wished.
5. Serve the chilli on warm plates, accompanied by the hot,
cooked rice.

Points per serving: 4.5
Total Points per recipe: 18

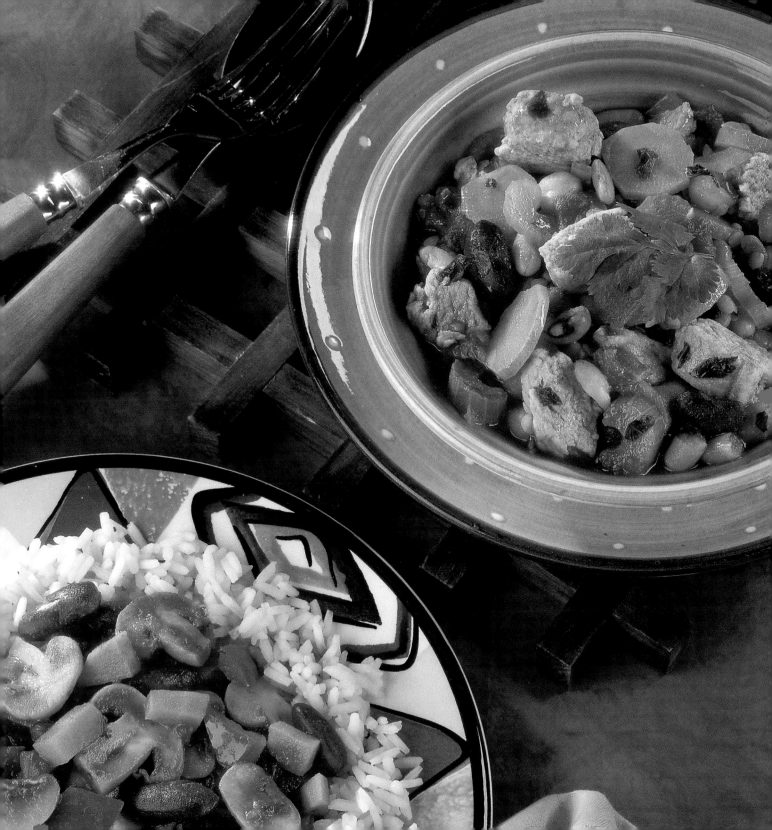

Salads

Some people think that anyone trying to lose weight must live on nothing but salads. Just leafing through this book would prove to them that this definitely is not the case! Salads do contribute an important part to our meals, supplying colour, taste and texture. However, it's worth realising that salads aren't always as innocent as they look. A coleslaw or potato salad becomes very fattening once a rich mayonnaise dressing is added, as do lettuce leaves when drizzled with olive oil. So beware, and prepare your salads with due care and attention. Follow the recipes given here to keep your salads low in Calories, yet very high in flavour.

Coleslaw

Serves 4

Preparation time: 15 minutes
Calories per serving: 85

Freezing: not recommended

Low-fat natural yogurt and low-Calorie mayonnaise give this crunchy coleslaw a lighter, easier-on-the-waistline dressing.

5 fl oz (150 ml) low-fat natural yogurt
2 tablespoons low-Calorie mayonnaise
1 large carrot, grated
a bunch of spring onions, chopped finely
2 celery sticks, chopped
1/2 small hard white cabbage, shredded
1 tablespoon chopped fresh parsley
salt and freshly ground black pepper

1. Mix together the natural yogurt and mayonnaise in a large salad bowl.
2. Add the carrot, spring onions, celery and cabbage. Stir in the chopped parsley and season with salt and pepper. Toss together well to coat the salad ingredients with the dressing.
3. Cover and refrigerate until required.

Points per serving: 1
Total Points per recipe: 4

Cook's note:
If you wish, add 1 oz (30 g) of sultanas or raisins or 1 medium-sized chopped apple to the coleslaw. Points per serving and Total Points per recipe will stay the same.

Chef's Salad

Serves 4

Preparation time: 15 minutes
Calories per serving: 215

Freezing: not recommended

This is a brilliant recipe for a tasty main-course salad.

1/2 Cos lettuce, torn in pieces
1/2 small Iceberg lettuce, shredded
2 beef tomatoes, sliced
3-inch (7.5 cm) piece of cucumber, sliced
4 oz (120 g) skinless, boneless cooked chicken or turkey, sliced in strips
4 oz (120 g) lean boiled ham, sliced in strips
2 oz (60 g) Cheddar cheese, sliced
12 radishes, trimmed
salt and freshly ground black pepper
For the dressing:
4 teaspoons olive oil
2 tablespoons light malt vinegar
1 teaspoon wholegrain mustard

1. Arrange the lettuce in 4 salad bowls. Divide the remaining salad ingredients between the bowls.
2. Whisk together the olive oil, vinegar and mustard. Season with salt and pepper and pour over the salads.

Points per serving: 4.5
Total Points per recipe: 18

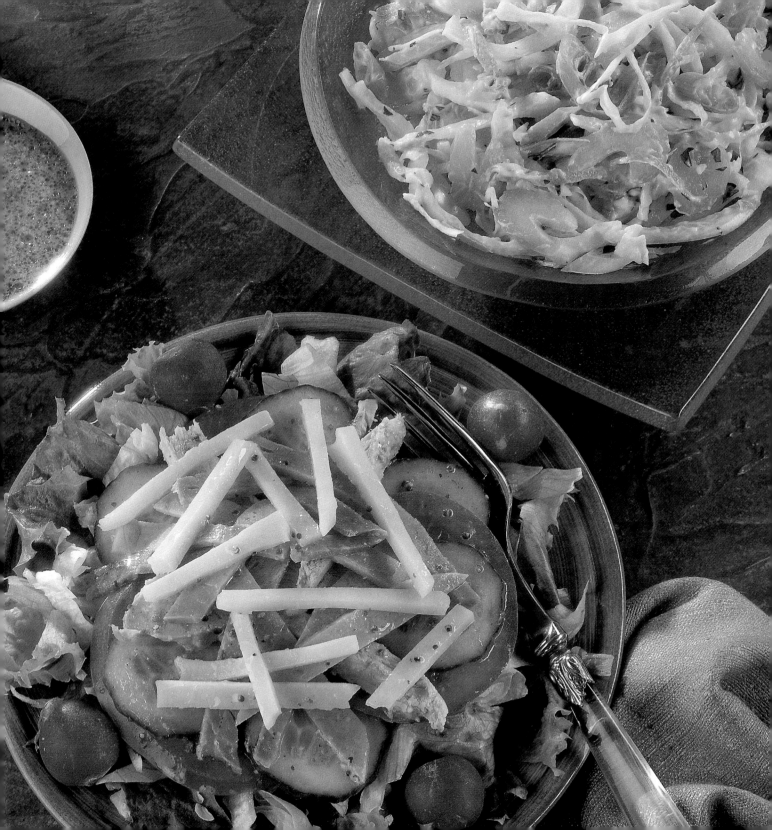

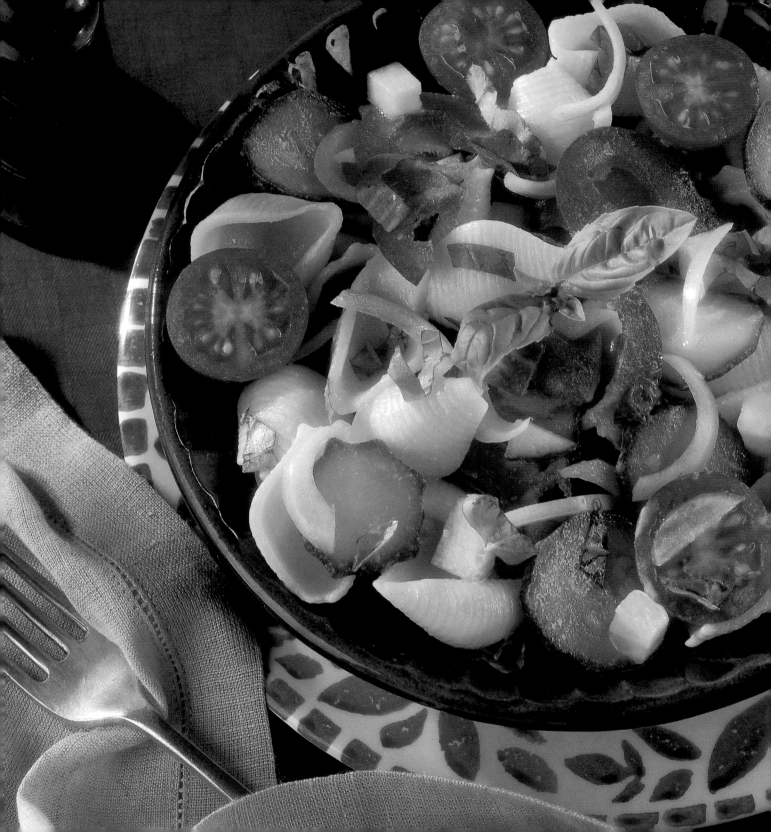

Pasta Salad

Serves 4

Preparation and cooking time:
15 minutes
Calories per serving: 205

Freezing: not recommended

Full of sunny Mediterranean colours and flavours, this salad will brighten any mealtime.

6 oz (180 g) pasta shapes
1 courgette, sliced

1 red pepper, de-seeded and sliced
1 small onion, sliced thinly
4 oz (120 g) cherry tomatoes, halved
3-inch (7.5 cm) piece of cucumber, chopped
salt and freshly ground black pepper
fresh basil or chives, to garnish
For the dressing:
1 tablespoon olive oil
2 tablespoons red or white wine vinegar
1 teaspoon French mustard
1 tablespoon chopped fresh basil or chives

1. Cook the pasta in plenty of lightly salted boiling water for about 8 minutes, or until just tender.
2. Meanwhile, cook the courgette in a small amount of lightly salted boiling water for 3–4 minutes. Drain and refresh under cold running water to cool quickly.
3. Mix together the dressing ingredients and season well with salt and pepper.
4. Drain the pasta and tip it into a large serving bowl. Add the dressing and toss well. Add the courgette, red pepper, onion, cherry tomatoes and cucumber, stirring to mix.
5. Serve, garnished with fresh basil or chives.

Points per serving: 3
Total Points per recipe: 12

Potato Salad

Serves 4

Preparation and cooking time:
20 minutes
Calories per serving: 110

Freezing: recommended

A great favourite gets the low-
Calorie treatment with a few
adaptations, and tastes every
bit as good.

1 lb (480 g) baby new potatoes,
  scrubbed
4 oz (120 g) low-fat natural
  fromage frais
4 tablespoons low-fat natural
  yogurt
6 spring onions, trimmed and
  chopped finely
1 tablespoon chopped fresh
  chives or parsley
salt and freshly ground
  black pepper

1. Cook the potatoes in plenty of lightly salted boiling water for
about 20 minutes, or until tender. Drain well.
2. Meanwhile, mix together the fromage frais and natural yogurt
in a serving bowl. Add the spring onions and chives or parsley.
Season well with salt and pepper.
3. Add the warm potatoes and toss them gently in the dressing.
Cover and chill until ready to serve.

Points per serving: 3
Total Points per recipe: 12

Cook's note:
If you can't find really small new potatoes, choose larger ones
and halve them after cooking.

Rice Salad

Serves 4

Preparation time: 15 minutes
Cooking time: 15–25 minutes
Calories per serving: 225

Freezing: not recommended

Use brown or white rice in
this delicious, colourful salad.

6 oz (180 g) brown or white
  long-grain rice
a bunch of spring onions,
  trimmed and chopped finely
1 green pepper, de-seeded and
  chopped finely
3 tomatoes, chopped
4 oz (120 g) seedless grapes,
  halved
1 oz (30 g) raisins or sultanas
salt and freshly ground
  black pepper
For the dressing:
2 tablespoons cider vinegar
2 tablespoons lemon juice
1 tablespoon chopped fresh
  mint or parsley

1. Cook the rice in plenty of lightly salted boiling water until
tender, about 20 minutes for brown rice and 12 minutes for white
rice. Rinse with cold water and drain well.
2. Mix together the cooked rice, spring onions, pepper, tomatoes,
grapes and raisins or sultanas.
3. Mix together the dressing ingredients and season with salt and
pepper. Pour over the rice salad, tossing well. Cover and chill until
ready to serve.

Points per serving: 3
Total Points per recipe: 12

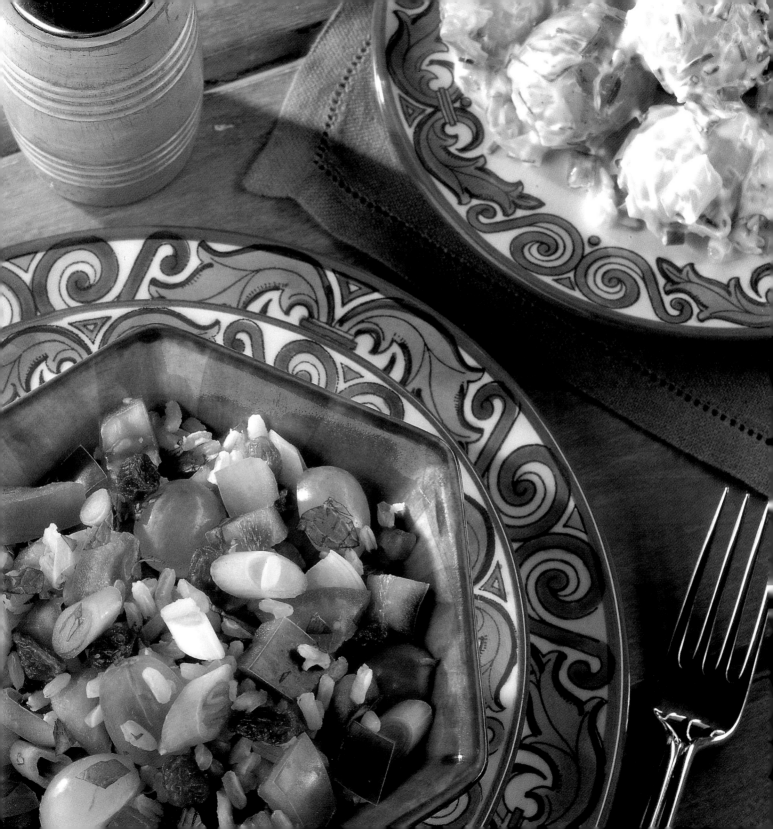

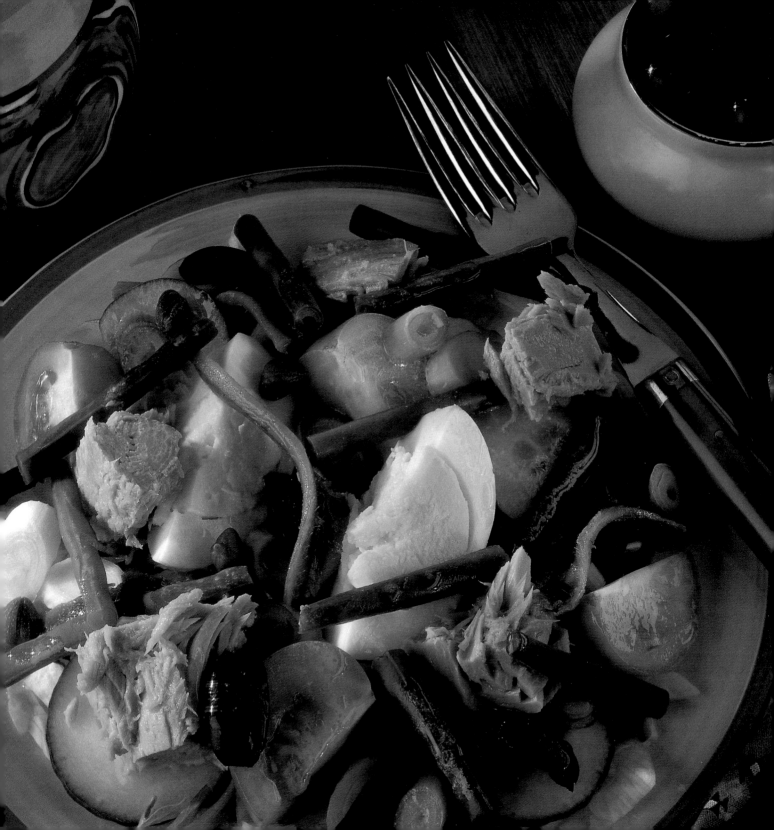

Tuna Niçoise

Serves 4

Preparation and cooking time:
15 minutes
Calories per serving: 185

Freezing: not recommended

A great storecupboard standby, canned tuna comes into its own in this all-time favourite recipe.

6 oz (180 g) dwarf green beans
¹/₂ Iceberg lettuce, shredded
4 small tomatoes, quartered
¹/₂ small cucumber, sliced
a bunch of spring onions, trimmed and sliced

7 oz (210 g) canned tuna in brine, drained
2 eggs, hard-boiled and quartered
6 large black olives, pitted and quartered
2 teaspoons capers
1 oz (30 g) canned anchovy fillets, drained and patted dry
1 tablespoon chopped fresh parsley
1 tablespoon olive oil
2 tablespoons light malt vinegar
1 teaspoon mild French mustard
salt and freshly ground black pepper

1. Steam the green beans for about 5 minutes, until just tender.
2. Divide the lettuce, tomatoes, cucumber, spring onions and cooked green beans between four serving plates. Flake the tuna and divide equally between the four portions.
3. Arrange 2 quarters of egg on each plate. Scatter with the olives and capers. Arrange the anchovies on top and sprinkle with the parsley.

4. Mix together the olive oil, vinegar and mustard. Season with salt and pepper and pour over the salads. Serve at once.

Points per serving: 2.5
Total Points per recipe: 10

Cook's note:
If you prefer, omit the anchovies from your salad and replace them with 2 oz (60 g) extra tuna. Points per serving and Total Points per recipe will stay the same.

Mixed Bean Salad

Serves 4

Preparation and cooking time:
15 minutes
Calories per serving: 135

Freezing: not recommended

**A very tasty oil-free dressing
adds flavour to this
marvellous three-bean salad.**

3 oz (90 g) dwarf green beans,
    trimmed and sliced
2 tablespoons lemon juice
1 tablespoon light malt vinegar
2 tablespoons tomato purée
1 tablespoon chopped fresh
    parsley or chives
a bunch of spring onions,
    trimmed and sliced
2 tomatoes, chopped
15 oz (450 g) canned red kidney
    beans, rinsed and drained
2 oz (60 g) bean sprouts, rinsed
    and drained
salt and freshly ground black
    pepper

1. Cook the green beans in a small amount of lightly salted boiling
water for 6–8 minutes, or until just tender. Drain and rinse with
cold running water to cool quickly.
2. Meanwhile, combine the lemon juice, vinegar, tomato purée
and parsley or chives in a mixing bowl.
3. Add the remaining ingredients to the bowl and toss to coat
with the dressing. Season well with salt and pepper. Cover and
refrigerate until needed.

Points per serving: 2
Total Points per recipe: 8

Caesar Salad

Serves 4

Preparation and cooking time:
15 minutes
Calories per serving: 125

Freezing: not recommended

**Try this classic salad with its
delicious, crunchy garlic
croûtons.**

1¹/₂ oz (45 g) anchovies in oil,
    drained well
2 teaspoons olive oil
2 tablespoons lemon juice
1 teaspoon French mustard
1 Cos or Romaine lettuce
¹/₂ oz (15 g) parmesan cheese,
    grated finely
4 teaspoons low-fat spread
1 garlic clove, crushed or
    1 teaspoon garlic purée
2 × 1 oz (30 g) slices white
    bread
salt and freshly ground black
    pepper

1. Soak up any excess oil from the anchovies using kitchen paper.
Mash the anchovies in a small bowl, and add the olive oil, lemon
juice and mustard. Whisk together and season with salt and pepper.
2. Wash the lettuce and tear the leaves into a salad bowl. Add the
dressing and parmesan cheese and toss well.
3. Mix together the low-fat spread and crushed garlic or purée.
Toast the bread on one side, and then spread the other side with
the garlic mixture. Toast again, and then cut in cubes. Sprinkle
over the salad and serve at once.

Points per serving: 2.5
Total Points per recipe: 10

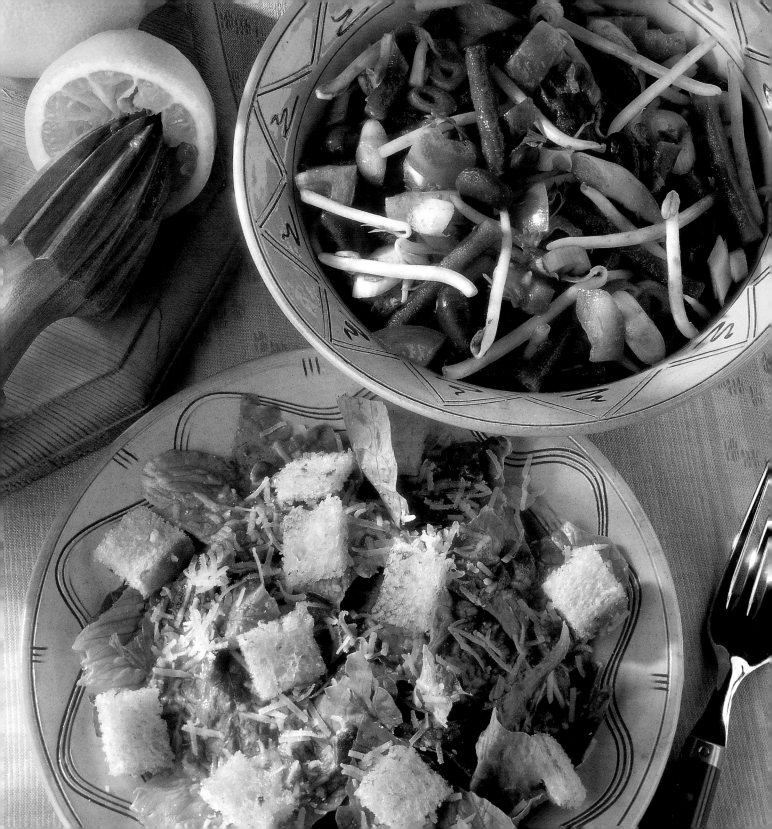

Desserts

Where do you look for that little bit of indulgence without going right off the rails? The answer is right here, with some delicious dessert ideas that will fit easily into the Programme. Just because a dessert tastes marvellous doesn't mean that it isn't good for us. Take the Summer Pudding (page 74) for instance. It is simply the most delightful dessert – a glorious construction of soft summer fruits, full of great tastes and fresh flavours. You would think that something that tastes so good has to be wicked – but not so! All of the recipes here take healthy eating into consideration, so enjoy your indulgence – free of guilt!

Bread and Butter Pudding

Serves 4

Preparation time: 10 minutes
+ 1 hour standing
Cooking time: 35 minutes
Calories per serving: 250

Freezing: not recommended

 If using free-range eggs

2 teaspoons margarine
6 slices low-Calorie bread
2 oz (60 g) sultanas or raisins
³/₄ pint (450 ml) skimmed milk
2 eggs
1¹/₂ oz (45 g) caster sugar
1 teaspoon vanilla essence
finely grated zest of 1 lemon

Simple, delicious and nutritious – no wonder this is one of our favourite desserts!

1. Grease a 2-pint (1.2-litre) baking dish with the margarine. Cut the bread in triangles and layer them in the dish with the sultanas or raisins.
2. Beat together the milk, eggs, sugar and vanilla essence. Add the lemon zest and pour over the bread. Cover the dish and let soak for 1 hour.
3. Preheat the oven to Gas Mark 4/180°C/350°F. Remove the covering from the pudding, and bake for about 35–40 minutes, until set.

Points per serving: 3.5
Total Points per recipe: 14

Rice Pudding

Serves 4

Preparation time: 10 minutes
Cooking time: 2 hours
10 minutes
Calories per serving: 140

Freezing: not recommended

1¹/₂ oz (45 g) short-grain rice,
    rinsed with cold water
1 teaspoon margarine
1¹/₂ oz (45 g) sugar
a pinch of ground nutmeg
a pinch of salt
1 pint (600 ml) skimmed milk

This is a no-fuss pudding that takes only moments to prepare, yet it always goes down a treat!

1. Preheat the oven to Gas Mark 4/180°C/350°F.
2. Sprinkle the rice into a 2-pint (1.2-litre) deep ovenproof dish. Add just enough water to cover the rice. Bake for about 10 minutes, until the rice has absorbed the water. Remove the dish from the oven.
3. Grease the edge of the baking dish with the margarine. Add the sugar, nutmeg and salt, stirring to mix. Pour in the milk and stir again. Sprinkle a little extra nutmeg over the surface.
4. Transfer to the oven and bake for about 2 hours, or until the pudding is thick and creamy.

Points per serving: 2
Total Points per recipe: 8

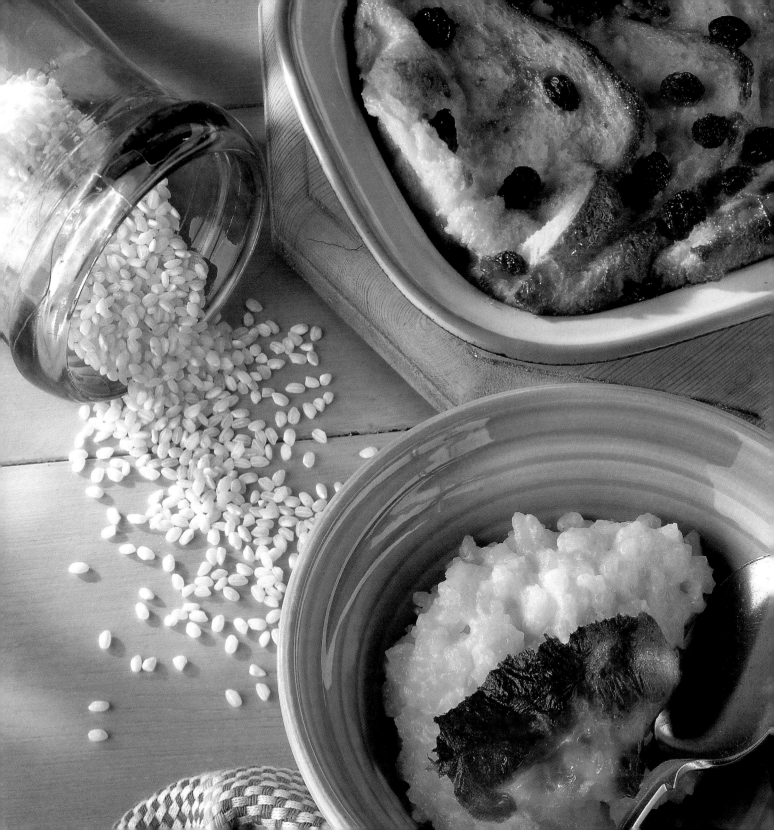

Summer Pudding

Serves 4

Preparation time: 20 minutes
+ several hours standing
Calories per serving: 140

Freezing: recommended

6 oz (180 g) blueberries
6 oz (180 g) redcurrants or
    blackcurrants
1 oz (30 g) caster sugar
6 oz (180 g) strawberries, sliced
6 oz (180 g) raspberries
6 slices of medium-cut white
    bread (4 oz/120 g in total)

**In this summer pudding the
bread is layered to make
assembly very easy.**

1. Place the blueberries and redcurrants or blackcurrants in a
saucepan and add the sugar. Heat gently until the juices just begin
to run. Remove from the heat and stir in the strawberries and
raspberries. Leave to cool.
2. Cut the crusts from the bread and discard them. Trim one slice
of bread to fit the base of a 1½-pint (900 ml) pudding basin.
3. Spoon half the fruit mixture into the basin. Press in half of the
remaining bread and spoon in the rest of the fruit. Top with a final
layer of bread, pressing down well.
4. Spoon any remaining juices into the basin to soak into the
bread, and then wrap tightly with clingfilm. Place a heavy weight
on top and refrigerate for several hours, or overnight if preferred.
5. To serve, turn the pudding out on to an attractive plate.

Points per serving: 3
Total Points per recipe: 12

Cook's notes:
Use any leftover bread to make breadcrumbs. Pack them in a
polythene bag and refrigerate or freeze to use later.

Use 1½ lb (720 g) frozen mixed berries instead of fresh fruit.
Simply defrost them and gently stir in the sugar.

Lemon Meringues

Serves 4

Preparation time: 10 minutes
Cooking time: 15 minutes
Calories per serving: 115

Freezing: not recommended

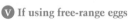 **If using free-range eggs**

3 tablespoons cornflour
¼ pint (150 ml) water
grated zest and juice of
    2 lemons
artificial sweetener, to taste
2 eggs, separated
2 tablespoons caster sugar

**You won't miss the pastry
at all in these delightful
tangy desserts.**

1. Preheat the oven to Gas Mark 4/180°C/350°F.
2. Blend the cornflour and water in a small saucepan. Add the
lemon zest and juice and bring to the boil, stirring constantly until
the mixture thickens. Remove from the heat and add artificial
sweetener, to taste.
3. Cool and then stir in the egg yolks. Make sure that the mixture
is sufficiently cool or else the yolks will curdle.
4. Divide the mixture between 4 ramekin dishes and place them
on a baking tray. Bake for 5 minutes.
5. Meanwhile, whisk the egg whites until they hold their shape.
Add the caster sugar and whisk again until stiff and glossy.
6. Pile an equal amount of meringue on top of each ramekin dish.
Return them to the oven and bake for 10 minutes, or until the
meringue is brown and crisp on the surface.

Points per serving: 2
Total Points per recipe: 8

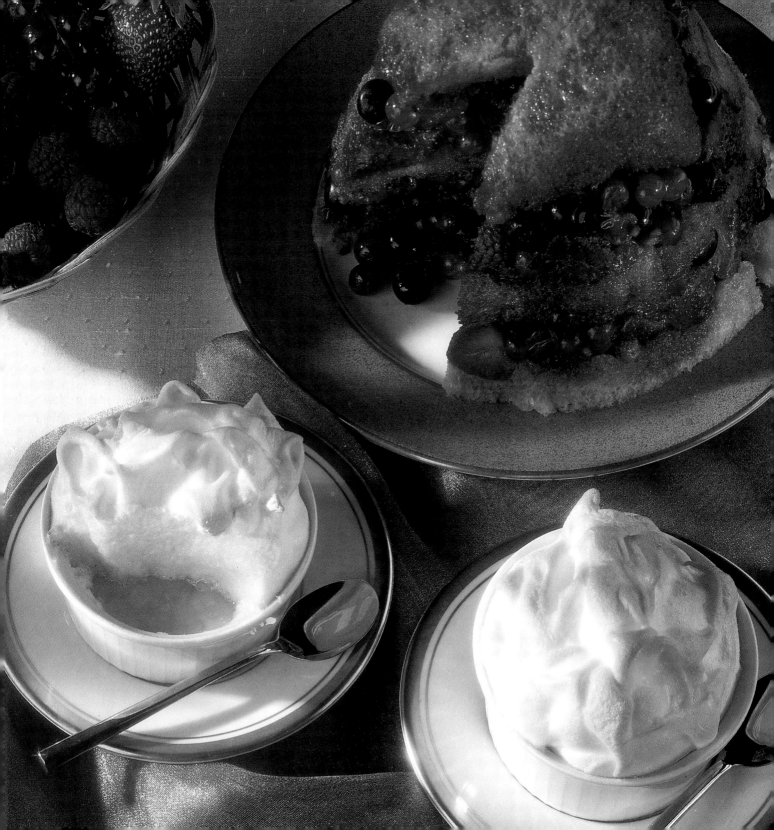

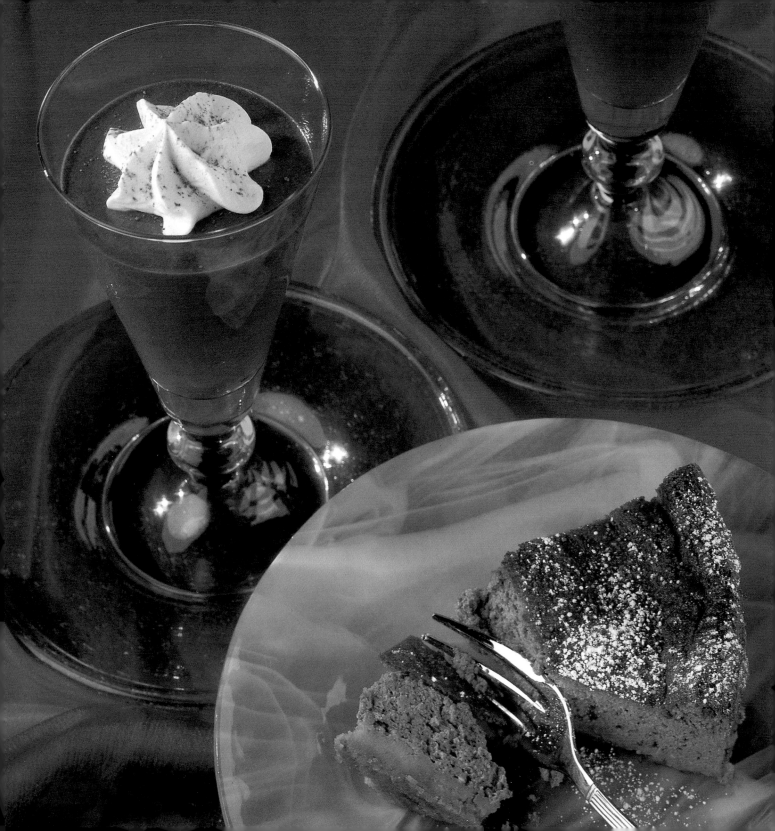

Chocolate Cheesecake

Serves 8

Preparation time: 20 minutes
Cooking time: 1 hour
Calories per serving: 195

Freezing: recommended

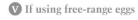 If using free-range eggs

Cheesecakes don't have to be difficult or time-consuming to taste superb – this one proves the point!

For the base:
3 tablespoons margarine
6 digestive biscuits, crushed

For the filling:
10 oz (300 g) low-fat soft
   cheese
5 fl oz (150 ml) low-fat natural
   yogurt
1 teaspoon vanilla essence
2 tablespoons unsweetened
   cocoa powder, dissolved in
   4 tablespoons of boiling water
artificial sweetener, to taste
3 eggs, separated
1 teaspoon unsweetened cocoa
   powder, for dusting
1 teaspoon icing sugar,
   for dusting

1. Preheat the oven to Gas Mark 3/170°C/325°F.
2. Line an 8-inch (20 cm) loose-bottomed cake tin with greaseproof paper or non-stick baking parchment.
3. Melt the margarine over a low heat, add the biscuit crumbs and stir to coat them evenly. Press them into the base of the cake tin to form an even layer. Refrigerate while you make the filling.
4. Beat together the soft cheese, yogurt, vanilla essence and cocoa mixture. Add artificial sweetener to taste, and then stir in the egg yolks. Whisk the egg whites in a grease-free bowl until they hold their shape. Fold them into the filling, using a large metal spoon. Pour the filling on to the biscuit-crumb base.
5. Bake for about 1 hour, or until set. Cool and refrigerate before turning out of the cake tin. Sieve the cocoa powder and icing sugar over the surface just before serving.

Points per serving: 4
Total Points per recipe: 32

Chocolate Mousse

Serves 4

Preparation time: 20 minutes
+ chilling
Cooking time: 10 minutes
Calories per serving: 195

Freezing: not recommended

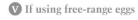 If using free-range eggs

Pregnant women, young children and those particularly susceptible to infection should avoid eating dishes containing raw or lightly cooked eggs.

2 oz (60 g) plain chocolate,
   broken in pieces
1 tablespoon unsweetened
   cocoa powder
1 tablespoon caster sugar
4 tablespoons hot water
2 eggs, separated
4 tablespoons whipping cream

1. Place the chocolate in a medium-sized bowl and place over a saucepan of gently simmering water until melted. Dissolve the cocoa powder and sugar in 4 tablespoons of hot water and add to the melted chocolate, stirring until smooth and blended.
2. Beat the egg yolks and stir into the chocolate mixture. Cook the mixture over the simmering water, stirring constantly until slightly thickened. Remove from the heat and cool for about 15 minutes. (To prevent a skin from forming, cover the surface with a circle of damp greaseproof paper.)
3. Whip the cream in a chilled bowl until it holds its shape, and then spoon half of it into a piping bag fitted with a star nozzle. Refrigerate until needed. Whisk the egg whites in a grease-free bowl until they hold their shape. Fold the egg whites into the chocolate mixture with the remaining whipped cream. Divide between 4 small serving glasses.
4. Decorate the desserts with piped whipped cream and chill until ready to serve.

Points per serving: 5
Total Points per recipe: 20

Cook's note:
If you don't have a piping bag, simply top each serving with a dollop of whipped cream.

Christmas Pudding

Serves 8

Preparation time: 20 minutes
+ overnight standing
Cooking time: 5 hours +
2 hours to reheat
Calories per serving: 210

Freezing: not recommended

V If using a free-range egg

**This fruity Christmas pudding
is absolutely spectacular –
likely to be the best you'll
ever taste!**

6 oz (180 g) seedless raisins
4 oz (120 g) currants
4 fl oz (120 ml) sweet sherry
½ teaspoon margarine
4 oz (120 g) carrot, grated finely
3 oz (90 g) fresh white
    breadcrumbs
finely grated zest and juice of 1
    medium-sized orange
1 teaspoon mixed spice
2 oz (60 g) dark muscovado
    sugar
1 egg, beaten

1. Put the raisins and currants in a bowl and pour enough boiling
water over to cover. Soak for about 20 minutes, and then drain
well. (This helps to plump up the fruit.) Add the sherry, cover
and soak for 6–8 hours, or overnight.
2. Grease a 2-pint (1.2-litre) pudding basin with the margarine.
3. Add the remaining ingredients to the sherry-soaked fruit and
mix thoroughly. Spoon into the prepared pudding basin. Level the
surface and cover with a circle of greaseproof paper. Secure a piece
of foil or greaseproof paper, tied with string, around the basin.
4. Set the basin in a steamer over a saucepan of gently boiling
water. Steam for 4–5 hours, topping up with extra boiling water
as needed. Never allow the steamer to boil dry, and always use
boiling water when topping up, to keep the heat level constant.

5. Cool the pudding once cooked, and replace the piece of foil or
greaseproof paper with a fresh piece. Store in a cool, dark place.
6. On Christmas Day, steam the pudding for 2 hours to reheat.
Alternatively, remove any foil wrapping and reheat the pudding in
the microwave on HIGH (100%) for 3 minutes. Allow the pudding
to rest for 3 minutes before serving.

Points per serving: 5
Total Points per recipe: 40

Cook's note:
This pudding can be made up to two months ahead and stored in
a cool, dark place.

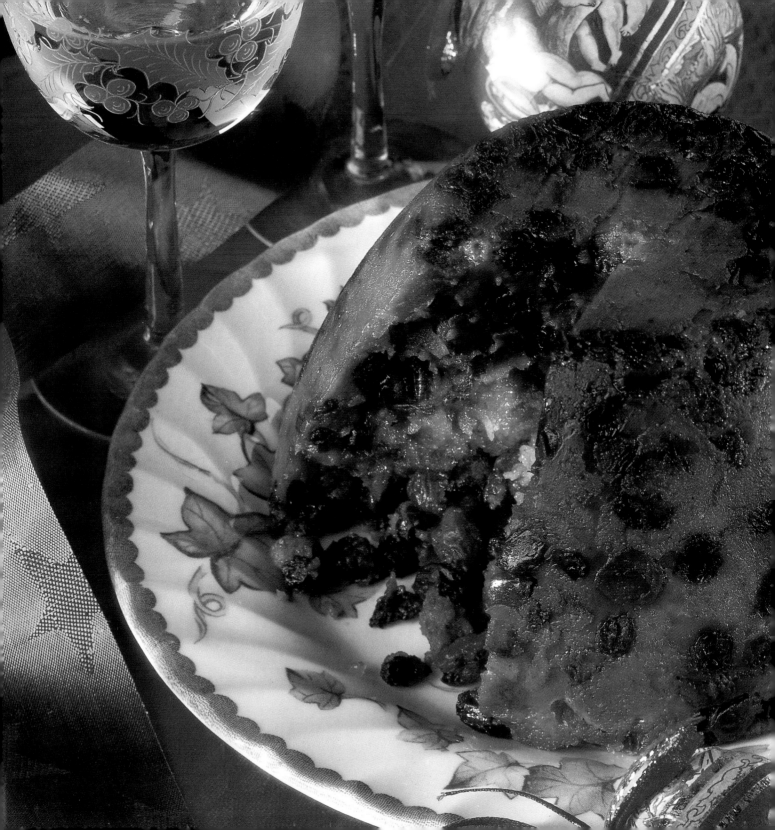

Index